Praise for *A Healthy Society*

"For those who seek the renewal of politics and public health in Canada, Dr. Meili has a vision for both. This work makes an important contribution to progressive dialogue in Canada."

Hon. Lorne Calvert
Former premier of Saskatchewan

"A very personal and passionate account from a doctor on the front lines of health care, this book should be required reading for every decision-maker in Canada."

Gregory P. Marchildon, PhD
Canada Research Chair in Public Policy and Economic History
Johnson-Shoyama Graduate School of Public Policy

"It is a huge privilege to be allowed into people's individual stories as a family doctor, to come face to face with their most private fears and challenges. To do so while seeing the bigger picture, learning what can be generalized from each individual story, is the finest way to honour one's patients as a physician. Ryan Meili has done this with *A Healthy Society*. His analysis shows that an understanding of health for individuals enriches our understanding of what Canada needs."

Danielle Martin, MD, CCFP
Chair, Canadian Doctors for Medicare

"A tour de force! In *A Healthy Society* Dr. Ryan Meili has interwoven the academic literature on the determinants of health with his experiences as a physician and community activist to present a vivid portrait of the adverse effects of current public policy directions upon the health of Canadians."

Dennis Raphael, PhD
Professor of Health Policy, York University,
and editor of *Social Determinants of Health: Canadian Perspectives*

"Dr. Meili makes a powerful argument: better health is a central narrative of our lives, our society, and our democratic institutions; so what's stopping us from walking the talk? A doctor's analytic eye diagnoses the problem: too much focus on treatment, not enough on preventing what makes us sick; too much focus on spurring economic development, not enough taking care of what we've got."

Armine Yalnizyan, CRC economist,
Canadian Centre for Policy Alternatives

"*A Healthy Society* is an eloquent cry from the heart and a rational appeal to the mind. With meticulous research, dramatic personal histories, and precise analysis, Dr. Meili shows why our wealthy society is far from a healthy one. He illustrates how social status affects physical well-being and suggests steps necessary to create a culture that's democratic not only in the electoral sense but also in providing for the health of its members."

Gabor Maté M.D.
Author of *In the Realm of Hungry Ghosts: Close Encounters with Addiction*

"Combining powerful analysis and compelling stories, Dr. Ryan Meili inspires us to engage in new politics to build a healthier, more equal society. May he continue to bring us together around bold ideas for change."

Niki Ashton, MP for Churchill, Manitoba

"Punctuated by moving and compelling stories from the front line of health care, *A Healthy Society* provides a brilliant exposition of the roots of good and ill health, and a much-needed vision for addressing the societal problems that keep so many Canadians from fulfilling their potential."

Gordon Guyatt, MD, MSc, FRCPC
Professor, Department of Clinical Epidemiology & Biostatistics,
McMaster University, and co-founder of the Medical Reform Group

A Healthy Society

A Healthy Society

HOW A FOCUS ON HEALTH
CAN REVIVE CANADIAN DEMOCRACY

Ryan Meili

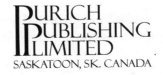

PURICH
PUBLISHING
LIMITED
SASKATOON, SK. CANADA

All inquiries and orders regarding this publication should be addressed to:
Purich Publishing Ltd., an imprint of UBC Press
2029 West Mall, Vancouver, BC, Canada, V6T 1Z2
Phone:(604) 822-5959 Fax: (604) 822-6083 Email: frontdesk@ubcpress.ca
www.ubcpress.ca
25 24 23 22 21 20 19 18 17   5 4 3 2

Library and Archives Canada Cataloguing in Publication

Meili, Ryan, 1975 –
    A healthy society : how a focus on health can revive Canadian democracy / Ryan Meili.

Includes index.
ISBN 978-1-895830-63-7

    1. Health — Social aspects — Canada. 2. Health — Political aspects — Canada. 3. Public health — Political aspects — Canada. I. Title.

RA418.3.C3M44 2012   362.10971   C2012-901444-3

Fourth Printing 2015

Edited, designed, and typeset by Donald Ward.
Cover design by Jamie Olson.
Index by Ursula Acton.

Purich Publishing gratefully acknowledges the financial support of the Government of Canada. Its book publishing program is also made possible through Creative Saskatchewan's Creative Industries Production Grant Program.

Printed and bound in Canada by Houghton Boston Printers, Saskatoon, on 100 per cent post-consumer, recycled, ancient-forest-friendly paper.

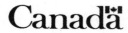

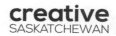

A Mahli
qui m'aime tellement bien

and to Doris
who told me to write a book

Contents

Foreword

HON. ROY J. ROMANOW

Former Premier of Saskatchewan

YOU HEAR IT ALL THE TIME — in the media, from the public, from politicians themselves: politics is broken. Canadians, and people around the world, are becoming increasingly frustrated with what they see as a widening chasm — a chasm between citizen values and public policy, between what people believe in and what governments do, between the world we envision and the one in which we live. There is a widespread belief, reflected in decreasing voter participation and growing cynicism among citizens, that the system isn't working as it should, that politicians aren't doing what they should. The question before us, as we hope for something better, is what exactly should they be doing?

For many years the primary measuring stick of societal success, and thus the primary goal of politicians, has been growth in Gross Domestic Product (GDP). By measuring economic activity, a growing GDP is thought to represent a thriving society. However, this measure is, by definition, insensitive to whether or not that economic activity contributes to the wellbeing of society. It counts things that harm us as well as those that improve our lives. The evidence against the use of GDP as a measurement is strong; it is clearly not a sufficient guide for our political actions. The problem facing policy makers, and disappointing the general population, is the lack of an accepted alternative.

Over the past decade or two, we've started to see the first signs of a significant transformation. There is, today, a growing international movement dedicated to re-defining individual and societal wellbeing in a way that goes beyond simple measures of economic consumption. The fact is that trying to gauge societal progress by using GDP alone is like trying to use a slide rule to measure blood pressure — it may give you a number but it doesn't tell you a whole lot about wellbeing.

Financial stability is an important element of societal success, a necessary tool for achieving our goals. It is not, however, the true goal of a society. As Dr. Meili argues in the following pages, a far more meaningful goal is that of health. Health — that of our neighbours and friends, our families and ourselves — is something we all seek. It's also a far better measure of success than material wealth.

For this wiser goal to take precedence, however, we need a change in government attitudes. Governments of all stripes have to view the decisions they make through the prism of "will it invest in the wellbeing of our society — in our health and overall quality of life — or will it diminish those things?"

A promising means of assisting that change in attitude is a new method of measuring societal success, the Canadian Index of Wellbeing. This project, led by a pan-Canadian group of research experts and practitioners, has begun tracking and providing unique insights into the quality of life of Canadians in eight interconnected categories that truly matter: our standard of living; our health; the vitality of our communities; our education; the way we use our time; our participation in the democratic process; the state of our arts, culture, and recreation; and the quality of our environment. In October 2011, the first complete, numerical report of the Canadian Index of Wellbeing, revealed that while Canada's GDP increased by thirty-one per cent in the period between 1994 and 2008, the quality of life of Canadians improved by a mere eleven per cent.

Aside from raising profound questions about the degree to which our economic prosperity is translating into better lives for Canadians, this report re-affirms earlier studies that demonstrate how closely linked wellbeing is to income and education levels. People with higher incomes and levels of education tend to live longer, are less likely to have diabetes and other chronic conditions, and are more likely to report excellent or very good health.

The stark reality is that household income continues to be one of the best predictors of future health status. The formula is straightforward: more income equals better health, less income equals worse health. This is true in all age groups and for both women and men.

When we consider the impact of this reality on those at the lower end of the income scale, we realize that there exists a vicious cycle: poor people have more health problems. They need more medical services, but they can't afford them so they cut back on medications or diagnostic tests, or they pay for them by cutting back on other things like nutritious foods. This leads to more illness and lost time at work, which leads to lost income and jobs, which creates more poverty. The end result costs us all — financially through increased social costs and health care costs, but also in our ability to enjoy life in safe, vibrant communities.

It becomes increasingly clear that if we are ever to break this cycle, if we are ever to significantly reduce the enormous health inequities that exist in our society, then we must address the full range of key determinants that cause those inequities — economic determinants, social determinants, educational determinants, health care determinants, and environmental determinants, to name just a few.

Historians tell us that we have had two great revolutions in the course of public health. The first was the control of infectious diseases, notwithstanding some recent challenges. The second was the battle against non-communicable diseases. I believe that the third revolution is about moving from an illness model to focusing on all the things that both prevent illness and promote wellbeing. This third revolution, in which governments and citizens work together to address the determinants of health, will ensure that Canadians are the healthiest we can be. It will also set the stage for Canada once again to be a world leader in innovation for better health.

The impact of the social determinants of health is well known to governments and to health care organizations. The major challenge before us lies in turning this understanding into concrete actions that have an impact on individual Canadians and communities.

Too often our understanding of the ways in which income, education, and other living conditions determine health status is not translated into the policies and services that will lead to change. We have not made the transition into a political system that creates the circumstances in which people can thrive, in which they can enjoy the fullness of wellbeing. Rather, there are many millions of people who continue to suffer from illness and die far too young due to the disconnect between our knowledge and our action.

The ideas confirmed by those who have studied the determinants of health, including the researchers who have developed the Canadian Index of Wellbeing, need desperately to be translated into the public pressure and political will required to bring about the third revolution in public health.

A revolution cannot happen without those individuals who are willing to take the risks to provoke lasting change, to turn ideas into action. If this third revolution is to take place, these leaders must articulate the vision of a healthy society in a way that people will find at once meaningful and motivating. Dr. Meili's experiences as a clinician give him an up-close view of the determinants of health in the lives of his patients. His passion for their plight brings a sense of immediacy to his cries for change. His personal experience, both political and medical, give him the outlook needed to propose practical solutions.

More than a voice for those who go too often unheard, *A Healthy Society* proposes a new approach to organizing for change. The stories of those most affected by the determinants of health breathe life into a reasoned argument for a system more responsive to their needs. The proposed focus for that system, the health of us all, offers us a common goal that everyone, regardless of their position in society, can support. *A Healthy Society* offers an inspiring means to fix what is broken in Canadian politics.

Saskatoon, 2012

Determining Health

The protection of the people's health should be recognized by the government as its primary obligation and duty to its citizens.

Dr. Norman Bethune[1]

A MAN AS THIN AS A SKELETON sits coughing in a tent near the hospital latrine, patiently taking his tuberculosis treatment and hoping he doesn't have a drug-resistant strain. A father's support makes all the difference for a young woman struggling to stay off of street drugs while waiting for cancer treatment. A five-month-old girl the size of a newborn is brought into hospital by her father, who has been feeding her canned milk since her mother died. An elderly man is sent to a nursing home an hour's drive away from where he's lived with his wife for 60 years; they can't manage at home with his dementia, and there are no long-term spaces available nearby. Having lost their home to flooding, a family wonders how it will care for a physically disabled child. A Dene elder goes into a diabetic coma and dies at home waiting for the ambulance that was busy with a car accident on the gravel road leading to her reserve. A doctor in a wealthy suburb prescribes an anti-depressant to a man who has been having trouble sleeping and concentrating; she wonders whether she should be taking them as well. Having lost his job due to an economic downturn, a middle-aged man is forced to choose between his children's school fees and his blood pressure medications.

Income, education, employment, housing, the wider environment, and social supports: these, far more that the actions of physicians, nurses, and other health care providers, have the most impact on our health. If Norman Bethune was correct, and the greatest role of government is protecting the health of the population, then it is in these areas that our public policy must have its greatest emphasis.

In *A Healthy Society*, the stories of patient experiences lead us into a discussion of health and its role in determining our political direction, our collective decisions. With health as a commonly held goal, the drive for better human health can be a shared mission for society. When people understand just what it is that really makes a difference in people's health — the determinants of health — it leads us to realize just how great a role politics plays in deciding the health of all of us. A renewed focus on health offers hope to change a political climate that has bred scepticism and mistrust among the public.

To begin, I will lay out the case for putting health front and centre in our public discourse — in how we organize politically, in how we plan, and in how we judge the success of our actions and our political representatives. In the following chapters, I will discuss the concept of social determinants of health in greater detail. Before doing so, I will pause briefly in the field of medicine and the health sciences to explore some emerging ideas that could be usefully applied to politics. We will then examine the current predominant focus for our society: that of economic wellbeing. This will be followed by the exploration of a number of specific health determinants, and end in a discussion of democratic reforms that could help reshape the way we organize ourselves to create a truly healthy society.

Chapter 1

A Healthy Society

The development of a society, rich or poor, can be judged by the quality of its population's health, how fairly health is distributed across the social spectrum, and the degree of protection provided from disadvantage as a result of ill-health.

Commission on the Social Determinants of Health
Closing the Gap in a Generation[1]

Buying Smokes for my Patients

Maxine just turned twenty, but walks like she's ninety-one. I suppose that's because she's closer to death than most ninety-one-year olds. You'd walk slowly, too, if that's what lay ahead. While she's been on the street since she was thirteen, hooked on IV cocaine and morphine for nearly as long, she has only had HIV for two years, three at the most. For some reason she, like many of the growing number of people infected with HIV in Saskatoon, is a rapid progresser. This means that, rather than taking years for her infection to progress to the immune suppression of AIDS, it happened very quickly. There are a few theories out there: different genetic capacity to respond, unique strains of the virus, or just poor underlying health. The truth is, we don't quite know why. What we do know is that she's in really bad shape — what many doctors would call, in back rooms and unprofessional asides, a train wreck.

When I first met Maxine, she came in with florid thrush, a rip-roaring pneumonia, and a prescription for prophylactic antibiotics she never intended to fill. I instantly recalled the hospital in Mozambique where caring for young men and women who arrive emaciated and scared, fast approaching the end of their lives, is a daily occurrence. Maxine's is the worst case of AIDS I've seen walking a Canadian street. I told her she was sick enough to go into the hospital, but she had just been discharged for the umpteenth time. She wouldn't say much, just told me she wanted antibiotics and nutritional supplements. The last thing she wanted was to go back into the hospital.

Three months later, the word on the street is that Maxine wants help. She's getting weaker and sicker, and finally recognizes she's in trouble. She comes into the clinic and falls asleep on the exam table. She is deathly thin, and under my stethoscope her lungs sound like a rubber boot being pulled from the mud. I call the Infectious Disease service and Internal Medicine at Royal University Hospital. They know her well; she's done this before. She gets sick enough to need some help, she is admitted, she gets a bit better, hates the hospital, misses the drugs, and bolts. Reluctantly, they agree to give her another try.

That was a Friday, and I was out of town for the weekend. When I arrive to see her on Monday morning the internal medicine team is about to discharge her. Her CD4 count, a measure of the immune cells that defend against infection, is four. It should be at least 400. The HIV viral load tells us how active the virus is in her system. More than 100,000 is considered too much; hers is three million. However, her pneumonia has improved, she's not ready for the antiretroviral medications that must be taken every day without fail in order to avoid increasing resistance, and the normal functions of an acute ward have been reached. She doesn't make it easy to help her, either. She swears at the nurses, refuses to take pills or have blood work. When the security guard assigned to keep her in line takes her for walks, she bums cigarettes, hides them in her gown and smokes them on the ward. She takes as much time and attention as the rest of the patients on her ward combined, and the nurses and medical staff are exasperated.

Despite her misbehaviour, she tells me she wants to stay. I visit twice a day, sitting on the edge of her bed and talking with her about the future. She says she wants to get on methadone and off the streets. She wants to take the antiretroviral medications to get her immune system working again. She is refusing to leave the hospital. The idea that, as health care providers, we might have security guards escort this young girl who is dying of AIDS to the street is against all we stand for.

So we don't. After a long discussion with the medical team, we agree to try a little longer. Give her a week and see how she does. Because, despite the frustrations of bed shortages, extra workload, and chances that are cachectically slim, we know these are the moments that define us as a profession. Even when the odds are long, we cannot walk away from someone who is so clearly suffering. So we'll try for another week. Get the methadone doc to see her, get psychiatry involved, and social work, and nutrition, and anyone else we can think of, make our boundaries clear and try once more.

We know the hospital is no place for Maxine. But the system has no better place. Most drug rehab programs won't take people on methadone; none of them will take someone who needs to start it. The waiting list to get started can be several months and requires people with numerous social and economic barriers to jump through multiple hoops that seem designed to keep them out. So in the gap between wanting to kick the drugs and having the personal and social capacity to do so, they're dumped back on the streets to start from scratch.

On the second or third night of this experiment in patience, I go up to see Maxine. The nurses are frustrated; she's still sneaking smokes into her room. She constantly demands that security take her for walks. She fights meds and blood work. But she's still there. She's taking her methadone. She tells me again she wants to stay, she wants to get better. The nurses think that maybe if she had her own cigarettes they could help her set a schedule and stay out of trouble. Maybe if they print her off more of the crossword puzzles she likes she'll stay busy. In many ways she is older than her twenty years. In others she's truly a child.

The next morning I go in to see her. I've got a couple of books of crossword puzzles and a pack of Player's Light. I never thought I'd buy a pack of smokes for a patient, but in this case "first do no harm" takes a back seat to the immediate fight for her life.

I go up to her room to deliver my gifts and talk to her some more. She's gone. The night before she got frustrated, left the hospital, scored some drugs, shot up and showed up in emergency in bad shape. The line was crossed and she is not welcome in the hospital any more. She can come to see me at the clinic the next week — we'll always see her — but the glimmer of hope is significantly dulled.

The last time I saw her, just before I stopped working at the clinic she trusts, she was repeatedly wearing out her welcome at the brief detox centre. I told her I hoped she'd at least come in and take her medications and see the other doctors there. She said goodbye, and thank you, and gave me a heartbreakingly innocent hug.

The cigarettes stayed in my freezer for a long time. I thought the next time I was invited to a sweat lodge ceremony, I'd bring them as my offering of tobacco and say a prayer for Maxine. It turned out I didn't get the chance — at least not while she was still alive. A few weeks after I left the clinic to work in rural Saskatchewan, she was hit by a car, shattering her pelvis. While in hospital she contracted pneumonia again, and this time she couldn't recover from it. She died just before her twenty-second birthday.

It's easy to get distracted by the pathology of Maxine's story, to think that it's a story of viral invasion, of fractured bones and infected lungs. These physical details, however, are distractions from the real disease. They are symptoms of what Dr. Stu Skinner, a Saskatoon infectious disease physician who specializes in HIV, refers to as the "End Stage of Poverty."

Maxine's life was hard from the beginning. She grew up in an environment of poverty, dysfunction, and abuse. Her mother had spent most of her own childhood in a residential school; she hadn't seen what it was like to be a parent and wasn't very good at it. Maxine never knew her father. Instead, she knew the attentions of various boyfriends and extended family members who abused her physically, sexually, and emotionally throughout her childhood. She had a baby before she reached Grade 9 and never returned to finish high school. In many ways she never got a chance to be a child, and at the same time never matured to be an adult.

Such a broken life, such an inherently tragic existence, provokes serious questions about our society: questions about the prevention and treatment of disease, about poverty and services for vulnerable people, about education, and about justice. What often escapes our attention when considering the tragic story of one individual is how intimately it is connected to all of us, to the collective decision-making process that is electoral politics. It is politics that decides whether young women like Maxine live or die. Ultimately, our political choices are to blame for the large number of people who slip through the cracks.

There is strong evidence that our current political choices aren't working for everyone. In Canada and around the world, the health of the poorest people is far worse than the health of the richest, and new evidence suggests we all suffer as a result. In order to address the fundamental unfairness of the situation, we need to rethink not just how we do health care, but how we make decisions as a society.

Economic growth and advances in health care have increased the life span, health status, and quality of life of people all over the world. Yet there are many people, in poorer countries and within wealthy nations, who do not experience the benefits of this progress. Canada is one of the wealthiest nations on the planet, but the gap between the rich and the poor is widening, and rates of child poverty and homelessness are on the rise. Despite Canada's self-image as a welcoming and equal nation, Aboriginal peoples, immigrants, and women continue to suffer more illness than the rest of the population. The cost of post-secondary education has risen to levels that are unaffordable for many. Epidemics of drug abuse, diabetes, obesity, HIV/AIDS, and other diseases closely related to poverty result in lost lives and wounded communities. Meanwhile, human actions are harming the wider environment that supports us; this, in turn, harms humans. These problems are fundamentally political, but those who raise objections to the current state of affairs, who suggest that there must be a different way of organizing ourselves that will be to the benefit of all, are dismissed as naïve and ignorant of economic realities.

None of this is news. Most people are well aware of the situation, and many are moved to action. The overall response, however, is fragmented, confused, and ineffective. The question before us all is, how can we move beyond this impasse? How can we organize ourselves to make wise decisions for the benefit of all?

Politics and public discourse, the field that should be responding to such pressing societal concerns, flounders instead from crisis to crisis. Parties and public figures bounce around the political and social spectrum in reaction to events or public opinion. The key issues of the day are decided more by the news cycle than any rational understanding of priorities. Ideas are presented by extreme opposite views in debate rather than in a search for common ground. Political reporting is dominated by scandal to the exclusion of substance, and, as a result, we are unable to focus on real issues. The agenda of governments seems to be either hidden or absent. From day to day the top stories change from an international conflict to a far-off natural disaster, from the rising or falling loonie to a record lottery jackpot, with no discernible pattern of progress or failure. In this fragmented experience of history and the present, all of us have a hard time recognizing what is really happening, what a government has done, or what it ought to do.

The problem is not a failure to understand the extent of our difficulties; it is the lack of a focus, of an organizing principle for change. An undeclared objective will not be realized; we must state our goals clearly if we wish to succeed in reaching them. In the absence of a societal project that advances the wellbeing of all, it is only natural that different groups will use politics cynically for their own gains, and that people will find it difficult to decipher the mixed and ever-changing signals. Without clear common goals, we have increasing polarity and discord. If we are to make anything of this mess, we must find something we agree on and work toward it. We need a clear objective that will inspire people from diverse circumstances to work together for a greater good.

What I propose is that people have already chosen that focus. It is simply a matter of recognizing, understanding, articulating, and acting upon it. The focus is health: the health of individuals, the health of communities, the health of democratic institutions.

People care about health. It's part of our assumed common ground, a truly shared value that transcends class, colour, and political ideology. Our conversations are replete with references to health. If you ask expectant parents if they're having a boy or a girl, the answer is inevitably, "We don't care, as long as it's healthy." When neighbours and friends are ill, we go out of our way to help them. If people fall on hard times, a common encouragement is, "At least you have your health." We speak of healthy relationships, healthy attitudes, healthy economies, and healthy appetites. We toast one another's health. These familiar expressions reflect our unconscious preoccupation with our common vulnerabilities, hopes, and fears: we know, deeply, that health — physical, mental, and social — is a necessary condition for the full enjoyment of life.

This focus on health is reflected in public life as well as private, particularly in the heated political debates around health care and health spending. Health care and health are very different things, but health care is the policy area most obviously linked to health, and the attention given to it is an identifiable surrogate for this deeper preoccupation. With rare exceptions, health care is the number one issue of importance in Canadian polling, an unusual constant in the tumultuous sea of public opinion. Accordingly, health care spending takes up the largest portion of provincial budgets. There have been many who have complained about this, saying that an inordinate focus on health takes away from other important areas such as education, justice, and infrastructure spending. In a way they're right — our focus on health care at the expense of other important aspects of public life is disproportionate. But the problem is not that we care too much about health, it's that we are doing so in an incomplete and reactive fashion. Our approach tends to be palliative rather than preventative; we focus too much on what to do when our health fails, not on how to make sure the conditions are in place for more people to thrive, to stay healthy. If we truly want a healthy society, we need to build a political movement with health as its focus.

So Urban it's Rural

To explore the idea of health as a focus for public discourse, I'll start with an example, one that for me hits very close to home. I live in Saskatoon, a city of nearly a quarter million people on the Canadian prairie. My house is in a neighbourhood called Riversdale, a few blocks west of the South Saskatchewan River. Riversdale is one of five core neighbourhoods that make up this area of Saskatoon, often referred to simply as the west side. Some people are surprised that a place the size of Saskatoon should have an inner-city, but it certainly does, with all its accompanying charms and difficulties. My neighbours keep an eye on the house when I'm away, and in summer they share fresh carrots and zucchini from their gardens. Strangers lean over the hedge to chat when I'm out raking leaves. People say "Hi, Doc" when we pass on the street. I often say it's so urban it's rural.

While its isolation amid the city's donut development (with peripheral suburbs and big box stores pulling social and economic activity away from the city centre) has conferred upon it some small town charms, its problems are decidedly urban. These neighbourhoods have the lowest per-capita income in the city. They have a reputation for petty and violent crime, and are the city's active marketplace for illicit drugs and prostitution. They also face a significant deficit in services, including frequent shortages of quality housing, access to good nutrition (there has been no real grocery store in the area for years), health services, and more. As a result, the health of the people who live in these neighbourhoods is the worst in the city.

Typical of the way in which these communities have been treated is the story of Station 20 West. In the spring of 2007 the government of Saskatchewan dedicated $8 million dollars to this innovative project, a collaboration between community groups in the core neighbourhoods, with the goal of addressing service gaps and creating economic opportunities. Community-based organizations such as CHEP (the Child Hunger and Education Project), and Quint (a housing co-operative based in the five core neighbourhoods) joined with the Saskatoon Community Clinic, the University of Saskatchewan, and the Saskatoon Health Region to design this unique response. The name, Station 20 West, played off its location literally just on the wrong side of the tracks crossing 20th Street, the core's main drag. It was billed as the Engine of Urban Renewal and consisted of a wide variety of services and community development initiatives in one convenient location.

Station 20 West was to be located next to 56 new affordable housing units and a branch of the public library, and was to include a dental outreach clinic, a community health clinic, a student-run after-hours clinic, offices for the aforementioned community-based organizations and others (including Heifer International and the Elizabeth Fry Society), a university outreach education centre, and a member-owned co-operative grocery store called the Good Food Junction. These were all to be housed in a building that would set a standard for environmentally responsible development with the highest level of LEED (Leadership in Energy and Environmental Design) certification.

At least that was the plan. In November 2007, the New Democratic Party (NDP) government was defeated in a provincial election and replaced by the Saskatchewan Party. In March 2008, the new government informed Station 20 West board members that the dedicated funds were being rescinded. Just months before starting construction, the project's future seemed extremely dim.

The new government's ill-considered decision to withdraw the funding for Station 20 West shocked the people of Saskatoon, triggering a firestorm of criticism and a groundswell of support for the project. In April 2008, in one of the largest demonstrations in Saskatchewan in decades, over 2,500 people from across the city took to the streets to proclaim their support for Station 20 West. Despite this show of support, funding was not reinstated, and the organizers had to start from scratch. Fundraising continues for a scaled-down version, without many of the earlier components. Over three years later, the much-needed services Station 20 West would have introduced are still largely unavailable.

At the time of this decision, I was working as a family physician at the clinic that was meant to relocate to Station 20 West. While working on the west side as a student, a resident in Family Medicine, and later as a practicing family doctor, I became quite excited about the potential of this project and was deeply disappointed by the cancellation of funds.

Clinical work in underserved areas offers many joys: the sense of community, the easy humour and relaxed attitude of many of the patients, and for me a sense of purpose, as I am often able to connect with people in real need and offer them meaningful support. The frustrations are many as well. Every day, whether I'm working in Northern Saskatchewan, rural Mozambique, or in my neighbourhood, I see patients whose problems are not merely physical, but political. They stem from a lack of safe or appropriate housing, a lack of education, or from simply not having enough money to access the basic necessities of life. People don't get sick when they come into the clinic or show up at the hospital; their problems can't be solved there, either. They get sick in their real lives: at home, at school, at work, and at play. Station 20 West was a project designed to meaningfully address the factors that play such an important role in determining longevity, illness, and quality of life: the determinants of health.

Healthy, Wealthy, and Why

The notion that health and illness are determined by life circumstances is not new, and in recent years it has become a staple of health theory and teaching. In one of the first lectures of medical school, students are asked what the greatest factors are in deciding whether someone will be healthy or ill. Lifestyle choices — like the so-called holy trinity[2] of diet, exercise, and smoking cessation — are a common response. Others will talk about access to health services, while others reference genetics or culture. After this discussion, the students are shown the list of health determinants from the Canadian Institute for Health Information. In order of impact, the factors that make the biggest difference in people's health are: 1. income status; 2. education; 3. social support networks; 4. employment and working conditions; 5. early childhood development; 6. physical environment; 7. personal health practices and coping skills; 8. biological and genetic factors; 9. health services; 10. gender; 11. culture; and 12. mass media technology (i.e., television viewing and physical inactivity).[3]

Invariably, this list is met with a degree of surprise. As aspiring doctors, the students think they are getting into the business of making people healthy. Then they see that the services offered by the health professions barely crack the top ten factors.

The lesson to be drawn from the list of determinants, and the one that is stressed to students, is that the most important factors that determine people's health are social, and the most effective solutions are political. Health services — the response to ill health — have much less effect on ultimate health outcomes than social determinants such as income and education, housing and nutrition. Gender, culture, and biology, the more immutable of the determinants, also figure near the bottom. What the students learn is that, while they can indeed have the power to heal, they cannot act alone. The response to illness is not limited to one profession or sector: it must be societal.

The question, then, is where does it make the most sense to focus our political efforts? In other words, which determinants of health are most directly affected by public policy? The social determinants of health are income and income distribution, education, unemployment and job security, employment and working conditions, early childhood development, food insecurity, housing, social exclusion, social safety net, health services, Aboriginal status, gender, race, and disability.[4] As you can see, these are all areas where public policy can change a person's situation or experience to either improve or worsen health. When we address inadequate housing, when we stop gender discrimination and racism, when we ensure people have access to work that is safe and fair and that our children receive the care and attention they need to grow, then we can dramatically improve health outcomes. So what's holding us back?

An Unhealthy Imbalance

The list of social determinants rings true to me and to others who work with the people of Saskatoon's west side. The majority of our patients are First Nations or Métis. They face challenges in accessing education for themselves, and child care and education for their children. Unemployment, poverty, and dependence on an inadequate social safety net are endemic, in particular for women. Housing is expensive, and often crowded or unsafe. Health care services are limited, and difficult to access. Violence, racism, sexual exploitation, and substance abuse are only a few of the many symptoms of ongoing poverty and social exclusion. The list goes on, and the result is ill health.

The effects of the social determinants on health are readily apparent to those who live and work in underserved communities. They are also supported by studies such as "Health Disparity by Neighbourhood Income,"[5] a 2006 paper published in the *Canadian Journal of Public Health*. This study compared the health of the six lowest-income neighbourhoods in Saskatoon (according to Statistics Canada) with the same health indicators in the rest of the city. The findings were startling. People in the core are four times more likely to have diabetes, four to seven times more likely to get a sexually transmitted illness, and fifteen times more likely to have Hepatitis C. Those in the core also experience significantly higher rates of injury, mental illness, and coronary artery disease.

When the six poorest neighbourhoods were compared with the city's six most affluent neighbourhoods, the contrast was greater still. If you live in the core, you are fifteen times more likely to contract a sexually transmitted infection, fifteen times more likely to attempt suicide, thirty-five times more likely to get Hepatitis C, and thirteen times more likely to have type 2 diabetes than if you live in the suburbs. Children in the core are half as likely to have received their vaccinations. With all these increased risks, a core neighbourhood resident is 2.5 times more likely to die in any given year. The infant mortality rate is three times higher in the lowest-income neighbourhoods than in the more affluent neighbourhoods.

To get a sense of income ratios, the average annual family income in the six core neighbourhoods was approximately $30,000 per year, in the rest of Saskatoon it was over $60,000, and in the wealthiest neighbourhoods it was just under $100,000. Forty-four per cent of families in the core live below the low income cut-off line, compared with less than four per cent in the high-income neighbourhoods. People from the wealthier neighbourhoods are more than five times as likely to have gone past grade nine or to have current employment.

This landmark study demonstrates clearly the huge disparities in health in Saskatoon and the clear correlation to the social determinants.

Saskatchewan has a reputation for seeking equality, in particular with regard to health. It was the first province to institute what would eventually become Medicare, a national health insurance program designed to ensure that all Canadians would receive health care based on need rather than ability to pay. It is also a reasonably well-off province in one of the wealthiest and supposedly most advanced countries in the world. The discordance between perception and reality represented by this drastic imbalance in health has been a shocking embarrassment for Saskatchewan. It is, paradoxically, not particularly surprising. We know, and have known for a long time, that poverty is the greatest contributor to ill health. What is new about this study is the way in which it shows, in simple and clear data, just how significant that effect is in Saskatchewan. And the implications are clear, although politically inconvenient: one, poverty and inequality kill;

two, governments that stand idly by are complicit in every avoidable illness and premature death.

Waking up Democracy

This embarrassment and shock could serve as a wake-up call. It could help to refocus our political discourse on the real work of a democracy. Our job, as people who govern themselves, is to strive to do so in a way that is fair and good, that allows all to participate fully and enjoy wisely the good things given to us by providence. A functioning democracy is one in which the government, to the best of its ability, carries out the will of the people and takes seriously its responsibility to serve the best interests of all citizens. This democratic governance requires a number of things, key among them being that people be sufficiently informed to articulate their real needs, sufficiently empowered to present them as demands that can't be ignored, and sufficiently organized to see the process through to fruition. Put another way, a democratic society requires a shared notion of what is good and a willingness to find a way to reach it. That is not to say that in the presence of such a shared notion everyone would agree and work together in harmony. Democracy is the messy, argumentative, pains-taking art of navigating a common course among conflicting priorities; were it not, we could be sure it was because all voices were not being heard. Having some shared framework, some set of guiding principles to steer the course, can allow these conflicting priorities to be weighed by all in terms of what is best for all.

I mentioned earlier the importance we give, in private and in public, to human health. The World Health Organization defines health as "a state of complete physical, mental and social wellbeing and not merely the absence of disease or infirmity."[6] Each of us wants health for ourselves and our family. The role of government in a democracy is to work with the people to produce what they want and need. What better goal for a society than to ensure that all people enjoy true health — a state of complete physical, mental, and social wellbeing? And what better measure of the success of a government, and the society it represents, than the health of the people?

If we as a society address the social determinants of health — economy, education, the environment, and more — people will live fuller, healthier lives. This much is clear. If we are transparent in our intentions, decisive in our actions, and honest in our evaluation of the results, we will also foster a common purpose that deepens community, builds solidarity, and rejuvenates democracy. In short, we will have found a means to move beyond our fragmented, haphazard approach to governance to one that works.

Yet there will be those who object to such an approach. Change is hard, especially if there is a cost associated. If people don't feel they will benefit, they will be resistant. Any reasonable approach to building a healthy society, especially one informed by social accountability or social justice, means that improving conditions among the poorest in our society must be a top priority. The foundation of a healthy society must be built among those who find themselves at the bottom. This is where addressing the determinants of health will have the greatest impact.

There are many people who see the world through compassionate eyes, who understand social justice, and act altruistically to improve the world. However, many of us don't see the world that way; perhaps we don't enjoy the luxury of doing so. We look first to the needs of our family, to a little more enjoyment of our own existence. We operate out of rational self-interest, and support the politicians who reflect our world-view, who offer us a little more money in our pockets, or protection from the forces that threaten our peace and security. What we fail to recognize is that it is in the best interests of everyone, even those at the top, to improve the health of all.

Helping Some Helps Us All

Addressing the social determinants of health doesn't just help those most in need; it helps everyone, regardless of social position. This is why the concept is so important: everyone benefits. This approach can be used to reach across divisions of class, race, geography, or political affiliation.

The poverty and ill health of some affect us all. Poverty is a drag on the economy. When people live in poverty they are unable to participate fully in public life and the marketplace, and are unable to contribute to the common account through taxes. They are also more likely to require health services, fall into the prison system, or require social assistance. People who do not have decent housing or access to education are less able to participate in the economy as customers, workers, or innovators. As their health suffers, the costs are borne by taxpayers. Our jails are not filled with hardened criminals (at least not when they go in); the vast majority of crimes against property and people stem from poverty. Our safety, prosperity, and satisfaction with society are decreased by gross inequality.

In *The Spirit Level: Why More Equal Societies Almost Always Do Better,*[7] epidemiologists Richard Wilkinson and Kate Pickett present compelling evidence that the degree to which resources are unequally distributed has a significant impact on the health of everyone. Countries that are more equal, such as Japan or the Scandinavian nations, have much better health outcomes overall than less equal countries such as the United States or Britain. While the ill effects of inequality are greater for those at the bottom of the social ladder, the impact is not limited to the poorest few. Health outcomes follow a gradient of wealth: people with low income have worse health than the middle class, whose health is not as good as that of higher-earning professionals, and so on up the social and economic ladder. But even the wealthiest people in an unequal society are less healthy than they would be in a more equal society. Whether it is the stress of constant competition and jockeying for position, the threat of personal ruin, or the burden of a large, marginalized population on public services and the social fabric, there is something about the experience of living in a society with a vast gap between rich and poor that damages everyone's health, resulting in more mental and physical illness, shorter life spans, greater levels of obesity, and higher infant mortality for everyone. Less equal societies suffer more of the social problems that lead to negative health effects, experiencing higher levels of violence, imprisonment, illiteracy, and teen pregnancy.

Life in a more egalitarian country, on the other hand, benefits the health of everyone, from the least advantaged to the most successful. The editors of the *British Medical Journal* grasped the significance of these findings: "The big idea is that what matters in determining mortality and health in a society is less the overall wealth of that society and more how evenly that wealth is distributed. The more equally wealth is distributed the better the health of that society."[8]

Any serious attempt to address health disparities must therefore involve a plan to address not just poverty, but wealth disparity as well. This is not an easy idea to sell, especially not in countries that have a strong systemic commitment to inequality. One need only recall the "Joe the Plumber" incident during the 2008 US presidential election, in which the mere suggestion of spreading the wealth of society more equally caused a huge uproar. This shows the degree of influence held by those interested in maintaining the current level of inequality. But if the cause of ill health is, as the *Clos-*

ing the Gap report asserts, the inequitable distribution of power, money, and resources,[9] then any serious attempt to address health inequities must involve a plan to distribute resources more fairly.

The UN Universal Declaration of Human Rights states:

> Everyone has the right to a standard of living adequate for the health and wellbeing of himself and of his family, including food, clothing, housing and medical care and necessary social services, and the right to security in the event of unemployment, sickness, disability, widowhood, old age or other lack of livelihood in circumstances beyond his control.[10]

When hearing stories of people living in poverty, the response is often that they are poor because of their own bad choices. People who succeed in life are those with the drive, determination, and skills to get ahead; they are people who make wise decisions. Looking back at Maxine, there's no denying that she didn't make the wisest of decisions. The question is, could she have done differently?

To choose well, one needs to have had the chance — through good role models, through childhood development, through access to the basic necessities of life — to have developed some real wisdom. Maxine didn't choose the life she was born into, and that life didn't equip her to make better choices than she did. In fact — through poverty, abuse, lack of education, discrimination, and social exclusion — it worked against her at every step. It's hard to imagine anyone succeeding in her circumstances. While there's no way to make a system that can force people to make wise choices, we can work toward one where more people have the opportunity to do so. By making the social determinants of health a primary driver of public policy, we can develop a society where more people have the chance to succeed and to live better lives as a result.

Providing everyone the opportunity to improve their lives, to escape poverty and experience the fullness of health, is not just the right thing to do, but also the smart thing to do. It is a delightful coincidence that our future wellbeing depends not on our selfishness but our generosity, our sense of justice. The growing gap between rich and poor impoverishes us all, diminishing the quality of life for rich and poor alike. We in Canada consider ourselves a developed country, but to allow the gap between rich and poor to grow is to become less developed.

The dream of a truly healthy society offers us a shared goal with the power to reach across the differences that separate us. It allows us to connect with our neighbours in recognition of our common vulnerability and our common desire to live full and healthy lives. By systematically addressing the determinants of health, and continually measuring our success, we can do both what is right and what is smart. We can chart a path of meaningful progress. We can improve the health of people and of the political system at the same time.

CHAPTER 2

Medicine on a Larger Scale

Medicine is a social science and politics is nothing else but medicine on a larger scale.

Rudolf Virchow, 1848[1]

RUDOLF VIRCHOW WAS A PIONEER in the field of pathology. Every medical student learns about Virchow's node, a growth above the collarbone that signifies stomach cancer. At some point in their studies they are sure to be quizzed on Virchow's triad, the three changes within veins that can cause blood clots. What fewer students know is that, as well as being the prolific scientist behind these eponyms, he was also a prominent 19th century German politician, and one of the first to write in depth on what are now referred to as the social determinants of health. He was also one of the first advocates of public health, stating that physicians, because of their constant exposure to the unequal distribution of sickness and early death, should be the "natural attorneys of the poor."[2]

Among his writings was the introductory quote to this chapter, a justification for his dividing his time between his practice as a pathologist and his political involvements. The idea that politics is medicine on a larger scale is one that influenced me not only to become directly involved in the political process, but also to seek what political lessons might be gleaned from the diverse study of human beings that is medicine.

The history of medicine is often described through major discoveries that change practice: the advent of penicillin or insulin, vaccines, transplants, dialysis, new drugs and procedures that cure or manage illnesses previously beyond our control. As important as these technologies are, the skills to use them properly, often referred to as the art of medicine, has evolved significantly as well.

An Evolving Art

In the past twenty years there have been a number of major conceptual developments in that art, and, subsequently, in the way it has been taught, that are beginning to have a major impact on people's health. These include the focus on social determinants of health, patient-centred medicine, social accountability, and evidence-based medicine.

The first — and the most profound, in my opinion — is the understanding of the determinants of health described in the previous chapter. While this is an intuitively true concept, and one that was advocated even in the mid-1800s by Virchow and others, it has only become a major focus of health study in the past three decades. Uptake in mainstream medicine has been slower yet, but in recent years it has become a central component of training, and a topic of increasing importance in the profession.

The second is the concept of patient-centred medicine. Once (and still in too many clinics) the rule was Doctor Knows Best. The physician asked the questions he considered important, examined the patient, told them what to take to feel better, and sent them on their way. The result: frequent misunderstanding between patient and clinician, misdiagnoses, prescriptions for treatment the patient was unable or unwilling to complete, and patients allowing responsibility for their health to be the doctor's and not their own.

Today's doctors are being trained to FIFE[3]: Feelings, Ideas, Function, Expectations. They explore the patient's *feelings* about their illness, the fears, concerns or hopes that have driven them to seek care. They then ask what *ideas* the patient has about the cause of their concern, often a very helpful step as the patient may clue in on a diagnosis very quickly based on their own experience and research. Next, the physician assesses the effects of the patient's health concern on their *function* at work, home, or school. Finally, the *expectations* for the clinical visit are discussed, allowing the doctor to understand what the patient's goals are rather than assuming they are seeking a particular prescription or other course of action. Once this process is complete and the situation well understood, doctor and patient can work together to find the best course of action, be it medication, referral to a specialist, a follow-up visit, or simply reassurance that their symptoms do not indicate a terrible disease. This method may take a bit longer at first, but, as one of the generation of doctors who trained this way, I find it saves me a great deal of time and guesswork. I've also noticed that when conflict does arise with a patient it's usually because I forgot to FIFE and focused too early on my own conclusions. Studies of law suits against physicians have come to similar conclusions: while people are forgiving of honest mistakes, they're far less willing to overlook poor communication. The end result of a patient-centred approach is an encounter far more satisfying to patient and clinician, better diagnosis, and much greater likelihood of successful treatment.

One interesting result of this approach is that the definition of success has changed. We now talk about meaningful outcomes. When we know what is meaningful to patients and their families, we can know whether to move ahead with a difficult treatment, or spare the expense and discomfort. The guiding principle is to do what will make the most meaningful improvement in the patient's quality of life rather than a focus on cure rates, survival times, or adherence to strict guidelines. This humanizing approach, based on what is significant in improving people's lives rather than an insensitive numerical standard, is an important principle to remember when we discuss political interventions as well as medical.

A related change has been a shift from the doctor as autocratic captain of the health team, holding all the power and giving orders to be followed without question. More and more, doctors are training and working in interdisciplinary teams, understanding that each profession brings a different understanding and expertise. This collaborative approach results in better overall care for patients. One example of this is SWITCH (Student Wellness Initiative Toward Community Health), an interdisciplinary student-run clinic in inner-city Saskatoon. SWITCH offers after-hours clinical services and health promotion programming to the community, providing an opportunity for students from medicine, nursing, psychology, social work, pharmacy, nutrition, physical therapy, and more to work together in teams from the beginning of their studies. This sort of collaboration allows for better communication between health providers, resulting in better patient care.

The third important notion is that of social accountability. The practice of medicine, the care of the sick, has at its core compassion and attention to those in need. It has also been a profession dominated by social conservatism, economic self-interest, and maintenance of the status quo. The social accountability of faculties of medicine, as defined by the World Health Organization, is:

the obligation to direct their education, research and service activities towards addressing the priority health concerns of the community, region, and/or nation they have a mandate to serve. The priority health concerns are to be identified jointly by governments, health care organizations, health professionals and the public.[4]

This means going beyond the work of treating the sick to understanding and addressing the reasons they are ill. The Parable of the River is often used to illustrate this approach. Imagine you are standing on a bridge. A flailing, drowning child comes floating down the river beneath you. Brave soul that you are, you dive in and swim to shore with the child. Before you can dry off and recover another child comes floating down and you dive in again and bring her safely to shore. A curious crowd has gathered by now. Another child bobs into sight . . . and another . . . and another. People take turns fishing them out. It doesn't take long before someone asks the pertinent question: who keeps chucking these kids in the water? And hopefully they head upstream to find out.

A socially accountable health system is one that dedicates resources to where they are truly needed, up and downstream. It is closely linked to health promotion, prevention of illness, and the social determinants of health. The design of such a system is necessarily complex, as limited resources are available to balance the demands of prevention and care. The more dramatic and tangible interventions — treatments and cures that quickly turn illness into health — get more attention. The things that prevent those last-resort interventions from being necessary are easily neglected in budgets and in our daily lives. On the other hand, no amount of prevention and health promotion will ever eliminate the need for health care. We still have to fish the kids out of the river. This complexity in identifying the priority health concerns, and the means to address them, is what necessitates the involvement of government, health professionals, administrators, and, most importantly, the communities they serve.

The fourth major advance in medical thought, and perhaps the most significant in changing science and practice, is that of evidence-based medicine.[5] This term, coined by Dr. Gordon Guyatt of McMaster University, describes a paradigm shift in medical practice. For centuries, medicine was a highly developed apprenticeship. Doctors studied and practiced based on what their predecessors had done, anecdotal evidence, conjecture about how things might work, and in later years the recommendations of pharmaceutical salespeople. Clinical science — and, in particular, its standard-bearer, the randomized controlled trial —have allowed us to evaluate tests and treatments much more rigorously. Today's physicians are expected to have a working knowledge of the analysis of evidence and to remain up-to-date in their field. They are assisted by journals, websites, and other easily accessible tools (such as the phenomenal RxFiles,[6] a Saskatchewan government-supported program which offers unbiased analysis of medications based on cost, efficacy, and safety) to ensure that they have the best of science to assist them in the art of medical practice.

The analogy of the past practice of medicine and the current practice of politics is striking. Rather than on the best evidence, political decisions are made based on a polling of their popularity, ideology, and other sorts of best guesses of what might work. What is needed is a move to evidence-based policy. We need to develop the clearest understanding possible of our goals, our meaningful outcomes. We then must understand the obstacles to reaching them, and the actions most likely to have the desired effect. We need to use the best information and examples available to us in order to build a healthy society.

Just as every person is different, even from themselves at another stage in life, every country, province, or city, at any given time in their history, offers different challenges and opportunities. There is no set of universal policies, but rather a broad range of potential tools to be used at appropriate times. Most political disasters stem from the application of theory in the face of conflicting reality. There is, however, a process for selecting the right tool that can be applied in most situations.

Thinking it through

To introduce that process, let me return for a moment to the Health Disparity report. This landmark study that demonstrated the gross discrepancies between the health of Saskatoon's poorest neighbourhoods and the rest of the city was only the first step. The creative researchers responsible for this study didn't want to deliver such terrible news without suggesting how to turn the situation around. They went beyond the collection and interpretation of data to try to discover what could be done. They looked at dozens of countries, from Ireland to Japan, and policy changes that have been effective in addressing poverty and improving health in those contexts. They then published "Health Disparity in Saskatoon: Analysis to Intervention,"[7] with their recommendations of policy options appropriate to the Saskatchewan context that would result in improvements in health. They made forty-six recommendations, from short-term strategies for housing and income stabilization to long-term educational and employment initiatives. While this study was criticized for failing to focus sufficiently on local strengths, it presented some compelling arguments, and for our purposes offers an example of how evidence-based policy can be made.

This process can be divided into four key steps:

Study: Be it a health problem, a business opportunity, or a gap in educational services, the first step is to understand the extent and character of the situation. For this step to work, we must first understand what our goals are. Knowing that we intend to improve the health of the population by addressing the determinants of health gives us a base from which to choose what to study. The authors of the Health Disparity report identified the growing health concerns in Saskatoon's core neighbourhoods and used the available data to better understand the situation.

Plan: Having developed an understanding of the problem, the next step is to come up with a plan of action. This requires diligence. All options must be considered and weighed in the local context. Historical successes and failures, local values and attitudes, existing resources, and more must be taken into account. Perhaps most importantly, the people who will be affected by any change must be consulted in a meaningful fashion. This step is key, as the people who live in a situation are able to understand it much better than an outside observer could. They may recognize flaws in plans or come up with better ideas that will work locally. Neglecting this participatory element of planning has been disastrous for any number of well-intentioned programs.

Act: The plan as developed must be properly resourced and put into action. Special care must be taken to understand end-points (when an intervention is finished) or program sustainability (how to support an ongoing intervention). While perhaps the most straightforward aspect of a program, this is the living test. The plan must be sufficiently flexible to adapt to changing circumstances, misunderstandings, and resistance. The better the understanding of and commitment to the underlying reasons for the change possessed by both community members and those who act out the policy, the more likely it is that, when problems arise, they can be smoothly managed. Here, unfortunately, is where the health disparities story stalled. The recommendations were just that, recommendations. Without the political will to follow through, which requires involvement and commitment from step one, the evidence languishes unheeded. Governments need to be a part of the process from beginning to end, committing to a full understanding of how social determinants of health affect the population and implementing the policies that will make a difference.

Fortunately, while their recommendations have not been wholly acted upon, the committed researchers and health advocates behind the disparities study continue to push for greater equality. They have formed the Saskatoon Poverty Reduction Partnership (with representation from provincial and municipal governments, non-governmental organizations, churches, and academic institutions) and identified seventeen of the original forty-six recommendations that had broad community, government and business support, including measures to improve housing, educational and employment opportunities, and raise awareness of the social determinants of health. As well as doing the hard work of trying to implement these challenging recommendations across multiple sectors, the partnership is also developing an appropriate set of indicators to define and measure meaningful outcomes, which leads us to the final step in the process.

Reflect: No matter how brilliant the idea and how diligently considered its application, the result may not be what was hoped for. Or it may exceed expectations and require further investment. The key is for the evaluation to be transparent; successes and failures must be clearly examined and communicated. One of the major challenges of government is to receive proper recognition for what it has done well. The current focus is on failure: governments downplay it as damage control, the media and opposition try to expose it. Honest discussion of intention and result, owning one's plans and their results, would lead to greater respect on the part of the public, particularly if they are involved in the process from beginning to end.

There is an ongoing need for innovations in measurement to allow us to better understand both the underlying situation and the effectiveness of interventions. To again quote Virchow, "Medical statistics will be our standard of measurement; we will weigh life for life and see where the dead lie thicker, among the workers or among the privileged."[8] Understanding the social determinants, their effect on the population, and the means of addressing them will require creativity and dedication on the part of scientists and policy makers. Work is underway on many fronts, in Canada and around the world, to collect data on health inequality along with gathering evidence on the most effective means of making change. Commitment to an evidence-based policy process that is rigorous and transparent will allow those developments to take place.

One example of this work is the World Health Organization's Commission on the Social Determinants of Health, which outlines a global agenda for health equity through action on the social determinants of health. The comprehensive report, *Closing the Gap in a Generation*, outlines three "Principles of Action":[9]

1) Improve the conditions of daily life — the circumstances in which people are born, grow, live, work, and age.

2) Tackle the inequitable distribution of power, money, and resources — the structural drivers of those conditions of daily life — globally, nationally, and locally.

3) Measure the problem, evaluate action, expand the knowledge base, develop a workforce that is trained in the social determinants of health, and raise public awareness about the social determinants of health.

This remarkably far-reaching document goes on to explore each of these areas in detail, citing the relevant evidence and outlining the steps for addressing the key health determinants. It is an excellent example of a framework for evidence-based policy on a global level and required reading for anyone with a real interest in the social determinants of health.

As the *Closing the Gap in a Generation* report demonstrates, the concept of evidence-based policy combines well with the notion of using the determinants of health as a guide for public policy, be it on a national, provincial, or local level. The determinants themselves — economics, education, environment, and so on — are already the stuff of policy. At every level of government, there are departments tasked with addressing these issues. What is lacking is a framework from which to measure our success.

Human health — physical, mental, and social — is the canary in the coal mine of the health of our society. It is a proxy or shorthand measurement for a host of meaningful variables. Using the social determinants of health to guide our policies, and health indicators to judge their effectiveness, gives us a much-needed yardstick. It allows us to move beyond the "gotcha" politics of personality and the goldfish memory of the news cycle to a long-term strategy for real development.

Health for all, understood in its broadest terms, is an appropriate overall goal for society. It's what a democracy is for. Just as in medicine, there is no political panacea, no one-size-fits-all cure for what ails us. There is no prescription for change; there is only a process. We must work out our progress "with trembling hands." Using the best evidence and tools to address what really determines health allows us to move more effectively toward our goal. Measuring and communicating the results allow us to evaluate progress and change direction as needed. This is a rational and meaningful approach to public policy. This is how a healthy society is built.

CHAPTER 3

Growth and Development

Income is perhaps the most important social determinant of health. Level of income shapes overall living conditions, affects psychological functioning, and influences health-related behaviours such as quality of diet, extent of physical activity, tobacco use, and excessive alcohol use.

Mikkonen and Raphael, 2010
Social Determinants of Health: The Canadian Facts[1]

Income from Within

The road to Tevele is red sand and sloppy in the rainy season. The pick-up truck bounces in and out of ruts as we head thirty-some kilometres from Massinga to this out-of-the-way rural community, located between the ocean and Mozambique's national highway. I am travelling with Dr. Gerri Dickson, director of the Centre for Continuing Education in Health, and two teachers from that institution: Cipriano and Flávia, both of whom studied in Saskatoon as part of their teacher training.

The Centre for Continuing Education in Health has a long relationship with Tevele. The *núcleo*, a group of leaders selected by the various surrounding communities, meets regularly with staff and students from the centre to address the health needs of the people of Tevele. Over the years, they have selected malaria and HIV/AIDS as areas of focus, and have done various public education campaigns and research projects to try to improve prevention and access to treatment.

Núcleo members, many of them quite elderly, walk for miles to attend the meetings. While waiting for those who are late to arrive, we huddle around a fire built in a hollowed-out section of a large tree to take off the morning chill. After morning tea, a group of keen participants starts a raucous gathering song: "*a kama wasiya*" (time is running out). It's a classic, well known by the members, and people clap and dance, animating the meeting grounds.

Like the centre, I also have a long relationship with Tevele. On each of my previous visits to Mozambique, I've taken time away from clinical work at the hospital to learn more about working with communities to improve health. The members of the *núcleo* are now old friends, and each visit feels like a family reunion. In 2007, I spent an extra week in the community, holding clinics and trying to improve my grasp of Xitswa, the local language.

The visitors and *núcleo* members gather under a large mango tree to start the day's session. The sun comes out and warms us to the point of leaving our jackets in the back of the pick-up. Part of the opening of every meeting is the singing of the national anthem: *Moçambique, Nossa Terra Gloriosa*, an event that is taken very seriously. Everyone stands at attention, looks straight ahead and sings in a sombre voice. Passersby on the road to town stop and stand until the song is over. This time, halfway through the second chorus, the rain starts anew. This is no drizzle; it's a tropical, soak-to-the-skin-in-seconds downpour. Given the solemnity of the song, no one can run and seek shelter. We grin and bear it, watering pouring down our faces as we finish the final lines of the anthem, then run into the newly built community development centre to start our meeting. While the topic is, as always, the health of the community of Tevele, today we aren't talking about malaria and mosquitoes. We're talking about money.

The most important determinant of health, much more than access to health care, genetics, or culture, is income. The members of the Tevele health *núcleo* may not have read the latest research on the social determinants of health, but they see every day the way in which the amount of money people have access to shapes their wellbeing and longevity. Every one of them has lost friends and family members to preventable and treatable illnesses like malaria, HIV, and malnutrition. They see how it is the poorest families that suffer the most, see how for the want of a few *meticais* a child dies at home rather than reaching the hospital for treatment.

Income is a determinant of health in itself, but it is also a determinant of the quality of early life, education, employment and working conditions, and food security. Income is also a determinant of the quality of housing, the need for a social safety net, the experience of social

exclusion, and the experience of unemployment and employment insecurity across the lifespan.

— Dennis Raphael[2]

One of the younger *núcleo* members, Senhor Ronaldo, has not been feeling
well lately. He has been losing weight and having frequent minor illnesses.
His wife had left for South Africa a few years ago and last year she returned.
She died a few months later. Many people from the area go to South Africa
for work in the mines and other industries there. Coming home sick from
South Africa has become synonymous with AIDS. Ronaldo has worked
with the *núcleo*, educating local communities about HIV/AIDS and other
sexually transmitted illnesses. He knows very well he should be tested and
start treatment if positive, he knows that both testing and treatment are free
of charge, but despite that knowledge, he still hasn't gone for testing. This is
not procrastination; he simply can't afford the 50 *meticais* (about $2 CDN)
to make the trip in one of the battered Toyota pickups that go regularly to
Massinga. If he had some form of income beyond what he can grow on his
machamba (small farm cultivated by hand) he would be able to access the
care he needs. If there were more local income opportunities, perhaps his
wife wouldn't have had to leave for South Africa to make money.

Recognizing how important local sources of income are for their families and their community, the *núcleo* members have embarked on a program of economic development. With the help of Canadian partners and
a group of young people called *Zambo ni Zambo* (Xitswa for step by step),
they have begun a *machamba* and a carpentry work shop and have recently
started to raise chickens. With help from CIDA (the Canadian International Development Agency), they have built a new "centre of competencies"
for meetings related to the economic projects and storage of related materials. Proceeds from the project go to a common account to continue
development, with a portion going to individuals involved, depending on
the work they contribute. *Zambo ni Zambo* also works with another of the
centre's partner communities, *Basso*, on a sewing project and a bakery. The
underlying idea is to increase the capacity of the community to sustain
itself economically. This allows local people to have more access to gainful
employment and income for necessities such as travel for hospital care and
medications, simple household goods like blankets, and more varied food
than what they can grow themselves. It allows them to find this income
closer to home, decreasing the disruption to family life and community

health brought by migrant work. This goes step-by-step with the health promotion and disease prevention activities of the *núcleo*, as rather than waiting for help from outside, the people of Tevele start to take charge of their own development. In the long run, these efforts may prove to be what makes a real difference, helping people like Senhor Ronaldo and his family to do better economically and live healthier, longer lives as a result.

Stories like that of Senhor Ronaldo's bring home just how important economic opportunities are for health. From Mozambique to Canada and everywhere in between, economics is the primary practical human activity. The exchange of goods and services governs much of our everyday life. The economic success of individuals has the greatest influence on their health, far above biology, access to health services, or culture. That success is also a significant source of social stature.

I mentioned earlier that health care is always at or near the top of the list of public priorities. Its main opponent in vying for public concern is the economy. People recognize how important economic success is for physical, mental, and social wellbeing. The list of determinants of health is topped by income and social status, with the position in the economic hierarchy being the single largest factor affecting health. Income also determines many of the other determinants: the ability to afford child care or higher education, safe housing and good nutrition, leisure and exercise, and in many places access to health services. It is little surprise, then, that those at the top of the scale for wealth are there for health as well.

Means and Ends

Nor is it surprising that economic success, such a key tool for reaching our goal of health and wellbeing, can get mistaken for the goal itself. This is a dangerous mistake. When a tool for reaching our goals gets confused with the goals themselves, we lose sight of the end and chase the means. Our political structures seek not to improve economies in order to improve our lives, but simply to improve economies regardless of the effect on people. In this sort of environment, measures of aggregate success such as GDP growth, rather than finer-tuned tools directed to true wellbeing, are used to measure our success as a society. And in such an environment, where the inequality of the distribution of ill health and poverty is not considered, a small number of people may grow very wealthy and well while a far greater number languish.

Gross National Product counts air pollution and cigarette advertising, and ambulances to clear our highways of carnage. It counts special locks for our doors and the jails for the people who break them. It counts the destruction of the redwood and the loss of our natural wonder in chaotic sprawl. . . . Yet the gross national product does not allow for the health of our children, the quality of their education or the joy of their play. It does not include the beauty of our poetry or the strength of our marriages, the intelligence of our public debate or the integrity of our public officials. It measures neither our wit nor our courage, neither our wisdom nor our learning, neither our compassion nor our devotion to our country, it measures everything in short, except that which makes life worthwhile.

— Robert F. Kennedy[3]

This is by no means an original observation. For decades people have decried the inadequacy of aggregate measures like growth in Gross National Product, or its more commonly used consumption-based cousin Gross Domestic Product, to assess real progress. Because all growth is lumped together, there is no mechanism to determine whether society as a whole benefits from it. By looking only at monetary transactions, things which cause harm can be seen as positive contributors to the economy. So-called externalities, such as the depletion of finite resources, environmental damage, or offloading of costs to other nations, can be ignored because they have no immediate bearing on monetary transactions. To quote University of Toronto philosopher Joseph Heath, "Anyone who treats economic growth as an overriding policy objective is therefore guilty of committing a 'count the benefits, ignore the costs' fallacy."[4]

The need for a subtler and more sensitive measure of development is acute. The Genuine Progress Indicator[5] is one such measurement, and there is excellent work being done by the Atkinson Foundation on the development of the Canadian Index of Wellbeing,[6] a much finer instrument for the numerical assessment of various aspects of societal success. The first full report of the Canadian Index of Wellbeing was released in 2011, showing that despite an increase of thirty-one per cent in GDP between 1998 and 2004, the wellbeing of Canadians improved by only eleven per cent in the same period. The availability of this kind of measurement is a promising change in the way we evaluate the work of governments, allowing us to point to concrete measures and the specific areas that require attention. However, they have yet to gain real traction among the media and the general public. If we tie them to the natural common interest of health, perhaps we can find a way to focus more attention on these efforts.

A Better Pancreas

One of my first public efforts to make the connection between income inequality and health was in 2006, when I was asked to speak to the annual convention of the Saskatchewan New Democratic Party about SWITCH, the Student Wellness Initiative Toward Community Health. I was part of a panel that included a young entrepreneur and the publisher of a magazine for Aboriginal youth. The idea was for the party, then in power as provincial government, to celebrate the successes of young people in Saskatchewan.

At SWITCH, students from Medicine, Nursing, Clinical Psychology, Social Work, Physical Therapy, Pharmacy, Nutrition, Dentistry, Kinesiology, and more work together, under appropriate supervision, to provide after-hours care and health promotion programming in Saskatoon's core neighbourhoods. As well as providing much-needed access to care in this underserved area, it is an excellent service-learning experience for the students. They learn in a practical, hands-on fashion about the social determinants of health. Perhaps most importantly, they make meaningful connections with real people, taking these important ideas from the theoretical to the personal.

As a student, I worked on the establishment of SWITCH, and later spent a year as the project co-ordinator. The government of Saskatchewan was generous in supporting the program, coming on early with funding and helping us establish legitimacy. At the time of the convention our doors had been open for a year, and I was pleased to share some of the successes of the program with our benefactors. I spoke of the hundreds of students on the volunteer rolls, the many different services, and the dozens of community members who access those services at each shift.

But I couldn't leave it there, on a falsely positive note. The Health Disparity Report,[7] released only a few weeks earlier, gave evidence of growing inequality and the suffering it causes. One of the conditions we see every day at SWITCH, one that people in the core neighbourhoods are thirteen times more likely to suffer from, is diabetes mellitus. Diabetes is the result of the failure of cells in the pancreas to regulate blood sugar. Rather than a proper balance of the fuel that cells need to operate, they have levels that are damagingly high or dangerously low. The analogy to the misdistribution of resources in our society, and the resulting ill effects on our health, is compelling. Initiatives like SWITCH and Station 20 West, valuable as they may be, treat the symptoms of a much deeper imbalance. Just as the body needs an effective mechanism to ensure that the needs of all its parts are met, with no organs starved or overfed, society needs a mechanism to make sure resources are effectively and equitably circulated. So, tongue-in-cheek, I urged the premier and his party — by enacting policies to more effectively distribute wealth — to become a better pancreas.

Turning the Tide

Aside from the risk of sounding ridiculous, I was cautioned by some against this approach. Redistribution of wealth has become a dirty word, even among left-of-centre New Democrats. No one talks about it any more, they said. And they were probably right. We talk about growth and the benefits it brings for all, of how a rising tide raises all boats. But the truth is that, while no one was talking about it, a massive redistribution of wealth had been taking place right under our noses. A small number of people have been apportioned a percentage of the wealth unprecedented in this country. This is the kind of destabilizing growth that undoes development, a disturbing trend for all involved.

The fact is that history has a direction. In recent years there has been an overall upward trend in wealth throughout the world. The economies of most nations, with rare exceptions among the poorest countries, are climbing in real terms. You might conclude from this that people's lives, so dependent on material wealth, are getting better. And in many cases you would be right. Life expectancy is increasing across the board. Indicators of ill health, such as maternal and infant mortality, are steadily decreasing.

However, when we look a little closer at the data, a different story emerges. Life expectancy is like the GDP of health indicators; it gives us a sense of aggregate success or failure, but can miss pockets of change that go against the grain. Some people are, in relative or absolute terms, getting poorer, and that decrease in wealth is accompanied by an increase in ill health. This is true on the whole in the countries of Sub-Saharan Africa and some geographical outliers like Haiti. It's also true within nearly every nation in the world, in particular the most developed nations known as the G8. The rising tide has not raised all ships; it has swamped and sunk the smaller craft. Many are left behind or worse off, despite the overall growth. The whole may or may not be greater than the sum of its parts, but some parts do much better than others. The result for those excluded from economic progress is more sickness and worse health.

The province of Saskatchewan, where I live, is no exception on either front. Our overall wealth has increased significantly in recent years. In the mid 2000s, under the government of Premier Lorne Calvert, we went from one of Canada's longstanding have-not provinces — provinces that receive equalization payments from the rest of the country — to one of the haves. Saskatchewan was booming, and it was touted across the country as the economy to watch. It was one of the last to suffer downturns in the recent recession affecting economies around the world. The swelling tide has been a source of pride and hope for many.

But not for everyone. My neighbourhood was once known for low housing prices. Lots of rental space, much of it not of particularly good quality, but people could always find a place to stay. Then the boom hit Saskatchewan, and housing prices skyrocketed. Over two years (2006-2007) the average price for a house rose by over fifty per cent.[8] There is likely some truth to the observation that this was a correction of some undervaluing of property, but the shift was dramatic and sustained. Houses were being bought up for renovation and quick resale, for condos and conversions. Speculation and the home-buying rush pushed vacancy rates to under one per cent,[9] and rents went up drastically — in some cases doubling in a matter of months. This provoked drastic change in people's lives.

The Little Boats

There's a family that comes frequently to the West Side Clinic; we'll call them Lucas and Annie. Hardly a week goes by that I don't see them in for a medical visit or just hanging out in the waiting room. They both have chronic medical conditions; he's had some trouble with the law; they've struggled with addictions. They can be friendly and charming, and they can be absolute pains. One of their daughters, Jaelynn, got sick a couple summers ago. Nothing too serious, but it required some specialist visits and more frequent follow-up with our clinic.

That was the summer we first started to see a new kind of homelessness in Saskatoon. The shelters at the YWCA and the Salvation Army were always full. There were more tents in the parks by the river. And in the mornings at West Side there was a line-up for the waiting room because people needed to have a place to hang out all day when they weren't welcome in the shelter or at the house where they were couch-surfing. Lucas got picked up for missing parole and had to spend thirty days behind bars. With him unable to contribute, and rent getting raised, they lost their apartment.

Annie would get a room for a week at the Y, or they'd convince a cousin to let them stay on the couch for a few days. Despite being hobbled with arthritis, she'd walk for hours with Jaelynn each day in search of an apartment. When Lucas got out, they tried going to his home reserve, but the housing there and in the town nearby was full as well. Despite all this transience, they kept up pretty well with their own medications, didn't end up using again, and got Jaelynn to all her appointments. She was improving quickly, and didn't need any serious treatment. However, after a few months back and forth in temporary housing, Social Services decided that they were not doing a good enough job of parenting and Jaelynn was apprehended into foster care.

Aside from the madness of trying to help children out of poverty by taking them away from their parents, this story illustrates an essential point. While the newspapers were talking about Saskatoon's housing boom, many families were going bust. The truth is that when the tide rises, especially if it does so quickly and wildly, the littlest boats get swamped.

This type of story is distressingly common. Economic growth across Canada has not been equally distributed. The gap between the rich and poor continues to grow, with the top forty per cent of earners experiencing real increases in wealth, and the bottom sixty per cent actually losing income relative to thirty years ago.[10] Canada's income inequality is worsening more quickly than it is in our historically less equal neighbour, the United States. This has happened in Saskatchewan as well, with the wealthiest ten per cent of families earning more than the bottom fifty per cent combined.[11] With prices rising along with wealth, the purchasing power of the average family is falling despite economic growth.

This is not fair. It also costs way too much — in social services, in lost productivity, in lost lives. The question isn't whether we can afford to do something about it. We can't afford not to. The question is, what can be done? How can a government act to change this? It's hard for political leaders, caught up in the glitter of boom times, to put on the brakes. This is especially the case when the prevailing orthodoxy is that since growth is good, then more growth, faster growth, is ideal.

Opening the Toolbox

There is a vocal group of economic thinkers who claim that what must happen is for government to get out of the way. If we simply allow the rational behaviour of people seeking their own interests to run free, then we will all benefit. The invisible hand will sort it all out. It's a pleasant notion, this idea that if people simply follow their own desires everyone's lives will improve. Unfortunately, that is like trying to reach your destination by heading in the opposite direction. People following their own wants cannot meet everyone else's needs. Growth, unless deliberately directed, results in the concentration of wealth among the few and increasing poverty among the many. The hand of the marketplace is not only invisible, it is also blind. It needs the guidance of our goals as a society.

> What can politics do? it must first accept the responsibility of sovereignty and the supremacy of politics in deciding the allocation of resources and the direction of future development. Let the economists decide the application and costs of the directions chosen. Secondly, Canada can grow and be of value to the world and to itself only by being an independent, sovereign state, and it can do this only by the control of its own economy and politics.
>
> — Eric Kierans[12]

We need to change the way we talk and think about the economy. A shift away from measuring our societal success by purely economic criteria could allow us to do so. The economy is an essential tool for reaching our goals of full health for all, but it is not the goal itself. Once we realize that, once we put the economy in its proper place as a tool, once we treat it as neither a force of nature beyond our control nor our ultimate goal, then we can start to use it wisely. That opens up all sorts of possibilities.

Economic management has been characterized, with great variation in the degree of each, by two main approaches, laissez-faire *vs.* state-involved. The former is characterized by a lack of regulations and minimal taxation, the idea being that economies function best unhindered and that external corrections are inherently damaging; somehow, if trade were truly free, if the invisible hand was given full rein, all would be well. The latter assumes that, since the purpose of the economy is its usefulness as a tool to reach societal goals, society should take control; if we plan and design well, all will be well. It is characterized by subsidies and regulations, often determined less by economic purposes than by political ones as politicians seek re-election. In such a system where supply, demand, and consumer choice lose their corrective force, we see stultification of growth and innovation, rampant corruption, and economic decline.

As tends to be the case, when we are presented with polar opposites, the truth is somewhere in between. The worst systems have been those in which either approach was taken as dogma.

The principles to preserve here are:

1. allowing space for innovation and growth (and failure and rebuilding) in a way that encourages entrepreneurship and hard work.

2. creating a system that is fairly and usefully regulated, allowing for citizens and companies to participate confidently in the economy.

3. identifying goals for the economy beyond its own proliferation. This returns us to the notion of meaningful outcomes. Just as in patient care, if we are looking to build a healthy society, we must know what that means.

The economy is not just any tool. It's the principal form of interaction in public life, and much of private life. But it is not that life. The first suit jacket I ever owned was a hand-me-down I wore to my med school interview. It didn't fit me very well and still doesn't. But in the pocket is a piece of paper with a quote from the Renaissance physician Paracelsus that I hoped, and still hope, would guide me in my decisions as a doctor:

If the physician understands things exactly and sees and recognizes all illnesses in the macrocosm outside man, and if he has a clear idea of man and his whole nature, then and only then is he a physician. Then he may approach the inside of man; then he may examine his urine, take his pulse, and understand where each thing belongs. This would not be possible without profound knowledge of the outer man, who is nothing other than heaven and earth.[13]

Just as we are so much more than the mere workings of our organs, our lives are so much more than the workings of our economy. The World

Health Organization definition of health as full social, mental, and physical wellbeing seems to me an apt description of what our real goals are, our meaningful outcomes.

Having understood that we have health as our goal, the question is, how do we work with the economy to reach that goal? The economy is a tool to make our lives better. If it fails to do so, we're not using it right. How can we use it more wisely?

The evaluation of any economic strategy (be it intervention or observation) must include not only the question, "Will it work?" but also, "For what (and whom) will it work?" In what way will it affect the economy, and will that effect be in line with our real goal, a healthy society?

This allows government to take the most important step: to see the economy as the vehicle we use to reach our goals, and economic policy as the toolbox that is key to maintaining the vehicle. We must not be the proverbial men with hammers to whom every problem resembles a nail. This is where you get into trouble — when tax cuts or tax increases, privatization or nationalization, become the approach taken to every problem. The appropriate role of government in different industries at different times is one of active intervention or benign neglect. What is needed throughout is not a fixed ideology, but attention and intention, especially in times of growth. If we understand what we want out of our economy, then we'll know how to manage it. If we use the tools wisely and appropriately to produce meaningful outcomes for the needs of the time, then that management will be effective. If not, the vehicle begins to drive us.

The Case for Fairness: Poverty Costs too Much

I started this chapter talking about the impact of income on the other determinants of health. The converse is also true. With a little consideration, it's easy to see how education level, employment conditions, physical environments, and social supports have a great influence on people's income and social status. This is true for individuals; it also extends to society as a whole. The healthier people are — which is a function of the degree to which the determinants of that health are met — the better they will perform economically and the better the economy as a whole will perform. The Conference Board of Canada, in its 2008 report, *Healthy People, Healthy Performance, Healthy Profits*[14] outlines the business case for action on the social determinants of health. The report demonstrates how businesses large and small can improve productivity and organizational performance by addressing the social determinants of health for their own employees, profit by taking the social determinants of health into account when designing and offering products and services that address pressing needs, and contribute to the overall stability of the economic environment.

The great thing about efforts to address the social determinants of health by reducing poverty is that, as well as improving people's lives, they also have enormous economic benefits. Poverty itself is a drag on the economy. *The Economic Costs of Poverty in the United States* study (2007)[15] showed that childhood poverty had a downward effect of four per cent of GDP on overall economic health. In Canada, poverty is estimated to cost an increase of $7.6 billion in health care costs, a loss of $13 billion in income taxes and a loss of over $35 billion in decreased productivity.[16] These enormous costs stem from the fact that when people live in poverty they are unable to participate fully in public life and the marketplace, and are unable to contribute to the tax base. They also are more likely to be involved in criminal activity, which has direct costs (property loss) and downstream costs (lost productivity, prison costs). They also tend to use more publicly funded services such as health services and social assistance. A country where fewer people are poor will have a much better functioning internal economy. Business owners have more customers with more disposable income and a safer, more stable environment in which to work and invest.

This is a neglected aspect of what is needed to have a successful economy over the long term. Investments in physical infrastructure, in roads and other supports that are clearly necessary for businesses to operate, must be accompanied by investments in human infrastructure — in health, education, child care, housing, and nutrition. When we have a healthy, educated populace, able to participate fully in the economy, we all share the benefits. We spend less on social services and enjoy the benefits of enhanced productivity.

When we allow people to fall through the cracks, we all share the costs. This is the functional feedback loop of economic prosperity: at a system level, economic growth improves the health of people, healthy people improve the economy. At the individual and family level, just as income affects the other determinants of health, they, in turn, have significant impact on income. The more educated you are, the better your housing, the stronger your social supports, the more able you are to contribute meaningfully to the economy. Where things go wrong is when the system and individual levels don't meet. If some people get healthy and wealthy while others stay poor and sick, fewer people are able to contribute and more require assistance.

While the amassing of great wealth has an obvious appeal to those who are able to do so, it has a destabilizing effect on the society that makes them wealthy. Greater differences in income increase social distances. Cuts to health and education lead to increased social stratification and demand for social services. If these go unheeded as tax bases are eroded, crime increases, and is increasingly directed against the wealthiest. If this trend continues, you get political instability that threatens to disrupt the country, including for the wealthy. So rather than enjoying the benefits of hard work and good fortune, the wealthy find themselves living in gated communities, isolated from and afraid of the dangerous world around them. More equal societies, where the difference in fortunes between those at the top and bottom is a gap that could feasibly be crossed, are safer and more satisfying to live in.

It's not hard to show people the need for greater equality. They see the effects on individuals and society wrought by economic disparities. Wealthy or poor, many people recognize the stress such inequality causes in their own lives. The challenge is to find an acceptable means of changing the current situation.

Guiding Growth into Development

Take the central policy importance given to economic growth: Economic growth is without question important, particularly for poor countries, as it gives the opportunity to provide resources to invest in improvement of the lives of their population. But growth by itself, without appropriate social policies to ensure reasonable fairness in the way benefits are distributed, brings little benefit to health equity.
— *Closing the Gap in a Generation*[17]

Economic growth can be an effective tool for improving people's wellbeing. As the story of Senhor Ronaldo illustrates, where economic opportunities are few, as in Tevele or many parts of Canada, growth is exactly what's needed. A more active economy is essential. While distribution must be a consideration in times of scarcity, it is not nearly as important as finding more resources.

Once a certain level of economic prosperity has been reached, however, there are diminishing returns. When that plateau has been reached, real benefits in terms of outcomes that are meaningful to health and wellbeing are best produced by better organization in the distribution of the proceeds of growth. Redistribution is far more efficient and effective in addressing wealth inequality and the wellbeing of low-income families than economic growth. The challenge before us is how to make the transition to development, how to make growth work for us: slow it down, speed it up, or tame it for our real good rather than let us be pulled blindly along by it.

The pendulum swing between good times and bad, richer and poorer, sickness and health, is an accurate description of Canadian history, and a potential vision for the future. As a province that has traditionally been dependent on raw material and natural resource industries such as mining, agriculture, fossil fuels, and forestry, Saskatchewan is particularly susceptible to the ebb and flow of world markets. The same can be said for most regions of Canada. If prices for our goods are low, we do badly. If prices are high, we do well. Sometimes we do spectacularly well.

Boom times are like an illicit drug. They're exhilarating and exciting, but they come with serious side effects. People forget about high interest rates, farm foreclosures, and families walking away from mortgages in oil-rich Calgary in the 1980s. They forget that booms have always been followed in the past by busts, and fail to plan for what happens when the downturn comes. The boom is fuelled by policies that foster undifferentiated growth, without a plan for development.

We will be stuck in this boom-bust cycle unless we recognize the difference between growth and development. Just as a tree farm is not a forest, a quickly growing economy is not necessarily a developed economy. Growth is an essential part of the economy, just as it is an essential part of cells, the building blocks of life. Cells must grow and develop and differentiate. Unchecked growth — growth for its own sake, with no intention and direction — is cancer. Development, on the other hand, is when that growth is applied, serving to improve society and create opportunities for further benefits.

Paediatricians who examine a child aren't satisfied to know if they are advancing along the growth chart, increasing in height, weight, and head circumference. They ask the parents about the child's gross motor skills, like turning over, crawling, or starting to walk, and fine motor skills like grasping objects between two fingers. They ask how many words the child knows, and whether they understand the world around them through interaction and play. No one would be satisfied to see a child simply getting bigger without showing some evidence of development; why would we be happy with an economy that grows without being certain that what it's growing into is positive?

Positive growth happens when we take the gains from our natural resources and invest them. We invest them in physical infrastructure, to be sure, but, more importantly, we must invest in human infrastructure: in education, in health, in housing, and transportation. That will give us a healthy, educated population that can take the gains from boom times and convert them into stability.

We must also consider that booms are generally based on non-renewable resources, things that will run out. The bust may be inevitable; the next boom is not. As a medical student, I visited Uranium City in northern Saskatchewan. The once-thriving community of five thousand is now a ghost town. A beautiful high school and crescents of suburbs stand abandoned and vandalized, a monument to short-term thinking. The uranium is gone, and the people with it. It may be many years before it comes to this in other industries, but we can't plan our future on things that won't be around forever.

We should plan our future on what will keep. The momentum of boom times should be used to free us from the boom-bust cycle, to create an economy based on long-term sustainable development. The knowledge economy, educating the next generation of scholars, can create an environment for research and innovation. An energy industry based on inexhaustible resources such as sunshine and wind can expand markets, create jobs, and provide for our energy needs. These and other industries based on resources and services that are stable in both demand and supply need to be the backbone of an economy that can weather busts and properly direct the force of booms.

Closing the Loop, and the Garage Sale

In Saskatchewan, we export nearly everything we grow and import nearly everything we eat. We have productive land and a population too small to eat everything we grow. But we are only able to produce certain things, so we cannot meet the needs and wants of the population, meaning importation and exportation are inevitable. While trading is an essential part of our economy, however, the current situation is unbalanced. We export things we could consume and import things we produce. More pathological perhaps, our economy includes the export of raw materials that go through relatively minor value-added production (e.g., logs to boards, wheat to bread, livestock to meat) outside the province and are returned to us. The waste of profit and jobs, and the negative environmental impact of transport make a strong case for closing the production-consumption loop.

Promoting knowledge economies, sustainable development, and value-added production is all part of the move from a garage-sale economy to one based on sound financial planning. No one would recommend a family sell its furniture, appliances, and clothes as its sole source of income. Yet this is what we do when we rush to extract resources as quickly as possible. There's no plan for what to do when the cupboard is bare. Governments are often exhorted to run more like businesses. Wise businesses don't sell everything they have and hope for more to arrive. They diversify their investments, take calculated risks, and plan for the future.

A more apt analogy, given the responsibilities and relationships involved, is that of government as a household. A wise family seeks out sources of income, managing debt cautiously and investing in the future. They take care of themselves, they feed and clothe their children, and make sure they get the education they need. When something goes wrong, they seek help from available services and from social supports, the family and friend networks they maintain. In short, they address the determinants of health; they do what it takes to make their family as healthy as possible. Government should be an extension of this approach, managing the resources and laws at its disposal for the common good, and seeking at each turn to choose wisely for the health of the population.

Finding the Balance — Incomes to Outcomes

The most direct, and perhaps the most achievable and measurable, way of addressing the determinants of health is to focus on making incomes more equal. Roughly put, there are two main ways of equalizing societal wealth. The first is post taxes (progressive taxation), the second before taxes (increased income parity). While the latter is more attractive, as it requires less "taking away" of earned wealth, both are probably necessary to some degree.

One example of a toolbox approach to economic management, one that reaches for the proper tool at the proper time rather than a one-size-fits-all approach, is the proper use of taxation policy. Taxation levels that impede economic development are unwise. That much is apparent. However, the notion has been taken to ridiculous extremes, with taxes falling in times of rapid growth for short-term political gain, disrupting public services and costing us money in the long term. What we need is the intelligent embracing of complexity rather than blind adherence to ideology and the approaches of organizations like the Canadian Taxpayers Foundation, who act as though (as Prime Minister Harper famously stated in 2009)[18] all taxes are bad taxes, and all collective investment is a bad deal.

The fact is that most of us save money by paying taxes. Comparing use of public services to income, the majority of Canadian families use far more in public services than they pay in taxes. For example, families earning $80,000 a year use approximately half that amount in public services.[19] This is due in part to the progressive nature of our tax system, which charges a higher percentage of tax to those with higher incomes. It is also due to the bulk bin principle; the more you buy, the less it costs. Imagine if each of us needed to pay directly for health care, roads, fire protection, snow clearing . . . the list goes on and on. Taxes, properly used, are each of us chipping in a small amount to buy something we need at a far better rate than any of us could get alone. The result is a great bargain on things we really need.

Those who bemoan any taxation either misunderstand the system or represent the views of the small percentage who pay more than they get back. This, too, is a misunderstanding, as the wealthy, no matter how hard working or intelligent they may be, benefit from public investment as well. This may be directly through subsidies to profitable industries, or on a more basic level from public infrastructure, labour, and sales markets dependent on the rest of the population, protection from calamity and crime, and through access to the natural resources of the land.

Using this kind of language about collective purchasing power and improved health allows us to discuss taxation in an adult way, rather than getting caught up in false representations that paint taxes as a way of robbing individuals of wealth and freedom. It opens up space for the discussion of simple changes that increase fairness. For example, in most Canadian provinces, people don't pay taxes on the first several thousand dollars they make. This makes perfect sense for those who make very little, but why do those who make a great deal more need to be exempt from this amount of taxation? In Newfoundland the exemption was removed from high-income earners, allowing the lower limit to be raised and eliminating income tax for more people of low income. This helps raise families out of poverty and encourages people to rejoin the work force, which contributes further to economic growth and decreases government expenditures. This sort of creative means of redistribution through taxation is an effective means of achieving multiple goals: increasing equality, improving health, and contributing to the productivity of the economy.

With all of that said about taxation, however, the truth is that taxes, for historical and psychological reasons, are unpopular. No matter how reasonable it may be, it's difficult for people to get excited about having money they've earned taken away from them. That's one of the reasons to explore other ways of levelling pre-tax income. This can be done in many ways, including:

1. expanding training, education and work entry programs, particularly for people from marginalized groups;

2. implementing policies that decrease the cost of housing and nutritious food for low-income families;

3. helping people get off social assistance not only by ending clawbacks for people who find work while on assistance, but by enhancing support during the transition period to full employment;

4. ensuring through indexation that minimum wages are always sufficient to keep working people above the poverty line. This has an impact on rates throughout the wage-earning population, making sure that a working wage is always a living wage;

5. protecting or enacting fair labour laws to protect people's right to organize and collectively bargain for their wages and working conditions; and

6. facilitating community economic development, like the Tevele *núcleo* or Station 20 West, in communities where stagnant economic growth and lack of employment opportunities are the main barriers to income.

These are just a few ideas for how a wide-open economic toolbox, one guided not by ideology but by utility, can help us to move toward our goal of a healthy society. Using health as the measure of success rather than blunt instruments like GDP allows policy-makers to adjust wisely in pursuit of that goal.

This is not to say that economy is not important. Quite the opposite. Income and social status are the factors with the greatest impact on the health of individuals and populations. The economy is too important to be left to dull tools and outdated ideologies. Too important to be measured badly. Too important a tool for accomplishing our goal as a society to be confused for the goal itself.

As former Saskatchewan premier Lorne Calvert always said, without economic progress, social progress is impossible.[20] By the same token, economic progress that erodes the social base on which our prosperity depends cannot be sustained for long. Social progress is economic progress. When we work to build a healthy society, we are also working to build the economy that can sustain and enrich that society.

Chapter 4

The World Around Us

One afternoon at the West Side Community Clinic I'm handed a patient chart. There's a sticky-note on the front directing me to Room 5 and an introductory line from the triaging nurse: "Not doing well at school, mother wondering about Ritalin."

I knock and enter the room to see a slightly pudgy little girl playing with the otoscope. She has short, dark hair and pink rubber boots dripping mud on the exam bed. Her mother sees me enter and hisses at her: "Jessica, sit down!"

Jessica is eight, I learn, and has been struggling at school. She's had to repeat one grade already and is in danger of having to do so again. Her teacher says she's distracted in class — at times disruptive, at times simply disinterested. At a recent parent-teacher interview, she suggested that Jessica may have Attention Deficit Hyperactivity Disorder (ADHD) and should be put on Ritalin.

Jessica is the middle child of three. Elaine, her mother, is on social assistance, and living with her daughters in a basement suite in the Pleasant Hill neighbourhood of Saskatoon. They've been there for two or three months after leaving an apartment she could no longer afford when her former common-law partner stopped paying child support.

After that the family had to spend time at Mumford House, a Salvation Army shelter for women with children. They moved briefly back to the small town where Elaine grew up, then moved back to the city when her relatives could no longer spare the room. Through these transitions, the girls have had to change school three times.

Elaine feels fortunate to have found their current place, but is worried about whether she'll be able to keep it. The month before, during an early season cold snap, the furnace stopped working. The landlord didn't fix it for three weeks and the family had to resort to a fan blowing over stove burners set at high heat to keep warm. When he finally did get the furnace fixed he grumbled that if they were going to keep asking for repairs, the rent would have to go up. They are already among the twenty per cent of renting families in Canada who spend more than fifty per cent of their income on housing.[1] Some landlords provide substandard housing at rates that rise relative to the social assistance rates, ensuring that housing costs continue to squeeze out any money available for other necessities. Rent squeezes the food budget, making people choose cheap foods of poor nutritional value. It squeezes the utility budget, keeping people colder in winter. It squeezes out other necessities like a telephone, clothes, laundry services, never mind a few dollars for recreation or entertainment to amuse and distract from the dull desperation of poverty.

In the examination room, Jessica is a bit of a terror, climbing over everything and interrupting incessantly while I interview her mother. When I talk to her about school, however, she clams up. When I persist with questions about her teachers and classmates, she makes noises and faces and acts up even more. As a family doctor, the question before me is, does she need meds?

Ritalin — or, as it is properly known, methylphenidate — is a stimulant drug that, somewhat paradoxically, works to help speedy kids slow down and concentrate. It can be very helpful in treating kids with ADHD. Jessica's struggles at school are consistent with a child with this problem. Even in the presence of these behaviours — which, according to Elaine, persist at home — I'm reluctant to come to a diagnosis and prescribe a medication. Are Jessica's problems really the result of a neurological condition? Considering all the moving, and all the challenges at home, how could we expect a child to be performing well at school?

In a reasonable world, we would look first to resolve the problems Elaine and her family are facing before treating the symptoms with a drug. This is easier said than done. Perversely, it is often easier for governments to cover expensive, mind-altering medications than to cover families from the elements.

I give Jessica's mother some forms to be filled out by her and by Jessica's teacher to get a better sense of the extent of their behaviour concerns. I also connect her to the social worker on duty, and write a letter to social services advocating for increased help with income and housing costs. These are good things to be able to do, but they rarely have great impact. The system is not particularly flexible; it is designed to give the bare minimum for families to survive in poverty, not to help them get out of it.

A Balanced Diet

That same day Don Bouvier was in to see me at the clinic. He's a talkative fellow; I know when I see his name on my day-sheet that it will take a little longer than the usual appointment. With some people that can be a bother, but with Don I never mind. He's always got an interesting story to share and, despite some big challenges in his life, he has a pretty sunny attitude. When Don first started coming to see me nearly a year ago, he'd been a while without a regular family doctor and his Type II diabetes had got badly out of control. His sugars weren't being controlled with oral medications, and if things didn't change soon he would need to start injecting insulin. I worked with him on getting a new glucometer to test his sugars, adjusting his pills based on those readings, and discussed changes in diet and exercise that could help control his sugars. I also got him in to see a physiotherapist and a dietician to do some more in-depth planning around physical activity and healthy eating.

Following up in clinic, I was pleased to see his sugars had improved somewhat. He was diligently testing and taking his pills at the right time. Despite all of this, however, his diabetes still wasn't well enough controlled, and he was starting to show signs of kidney problems. Because he was already taking the maximum dose of oral medications, if the sugars didn't come down further, he would need to start giving himself injections of insulin. While that's not the end of the world, it's something most patients would like to avoid as long as possible. I asked him again about diet and exercise.

Due to serious injuries he got on the job as a young man, Don isn't able to work regularly. A single father, he takes care of two teenage sons and a nephew. He does some casual work when he's able, but is restricted by his disability. His main source of income is social assistance. His ability to exercise is limited; he walks everywhere he can, but can do little else without significant pain. As for nutrition, Don has no trouble telling me what he should eat and what he should avoid. He understood perfectly the recommendations from the dietician and has tried to make some changes, but this is where he runs into real trouble. He knows what he should eat but healthier foods are hard to find and even harder to afford.

As the city has grown in recent years there's been a shift in the location of food stores. Most of the grocery stores are now in suburban areas and are difficult to access without a vehicle. In Don's neighbourhood, there used to be two full grocery stores; both have now closed. Rumour has it these stores were profitable, just not at the level of suburban stores. There are convenience stores and a Giant Tiger discount store that carry some groceries, but these are dominated by pre-packaged foods and junk food like pop and chips. Fresh produce is limited and expensive, as are whole grain foods and fresh meat. Feeding three growing teenage boys food they'll eat while following a strict diabetic diet himself is simply beyond Don's means.

Don is one of many patients with similar stories. In inner-city neighbourhoods and in small towns, and especially in remote communities where the costs of basics like milk and bread can be astronomical, food insecurity is a concern for thousands of Canadian families. While sometimes the problem is a lack of understanding of which foods are healthy and which are harmful, more often it is a matter of affordability and accessibility. People want to eat right, but they don't want their families to be hungry. The truth is that on a limited budget, the bad food stretches further. In Mozambique, when we see children who are malnourished, it is obvious: they are emaciated, all skin and bones and sunken eyes. In Canada, the malnourishment is hidden under a layer of fat. Kids are not getting what they need to be healthy, to grow well, and to prevent illness. Instead, they are fed over-processed empty calories, high in salt and sugar — foods that are cheap, tasty, and harmful.

Hitting Where we Live

The determinants of health largely refer to a person's place in society — for example, their wages relative to national averages, the type of employment they have, the family and friends they can count on. These larger realities are hugely influential on our health, but they are in some ways abstract and less immediate than our actual places, our physical environments.

The most immediate of these physical environments is the homes we live in. Consider, with that, the places we work, study, and play, the food we eat, the clothes we wear, the water we drink, and the air we breathe, and you begin to get a picture of how inextricably linked our health is to the world around us. This is not a contentious assertion. You would be hard pressed to find someone who would argue that external conditions had nothing to do with the likelihood of experiencing illness.

Despite both intuitive and scientific evidence that supports the connection between where and how we live and our health, somehow improving these circumstances takes a back seat to other spending priorities, or to tax cuts. In Canada, despite reports from all levels of government on the need for comprehensive housing strategies, these same governments have been backing away from meaningful investments in social housing for decades. The most significant such change was the Canadian federal government's decision in the early 1990s to no longer build new social housing units. The argument is that the private sector will be more efficient and effective at producing housing.

The private sector excels at producing homes for ownership, or for high income rental property. Developers are good at this because it is the most profitable area of the housing market, and because their aim is to make profits for their owners and investors. Handing over housing strategy to the private sector in order to make housing affordable for low-income families is like trying to wash your dishes in the clothes-dryer. It's a useful appliance, but that's not what it's for.

The evidence from this experiment supports that scepticism. The numbers of available units has shrunk through condo conversion and the elimination of older rental properties, and the quality of available and affordable housing stock is deteriorating. This means that, despite stagnant wages, low- and middle-income families are paying more to live in worse places.

Those who aren't able to pay find themselves in a worse circumstance yet. Some couch surf. Others crowd into apartments meant for far fewer people, a condition referred to as relative homelessness. A growing number find themselves with nowhere to go. In large cities and small towns across the country, shelters are too full to accept everyone in need.

Our values as a society, and the harsh realities of our climate, make a growing homeless population unacceptable to Canadians. Advocacy organizations like Passion for Action for Homelessness, shelter networks such as the Out of the Cold church basement programs that operate in a number of Canadian cities, Anti-Poverty Coalitions and others continue to work to raise awareness, pressure policy-makers and fill the gaps where they can. Academics and advocacy groups, such as the Toronto Disaster Relief Committee, have proposed something they call the one per cent solution.[2] Prior to the 1990s, provincial, federal, and municipal governments spent, on average, one per cent of their budgets on housing. These groups describe how a return to those levels, properly applied with increased investment in social housing, increased rent supplements for low-income families, supportive housing for those in need, grants for improvement of existing housing stock, and, when necessary, temporary shelters for homeless people, could make the Canadian housing crisis far less damaging to people and the economies that support them. Recognition across the country of the need for change continues to grow, and the cry for a national housing strategy gets louder all the time.

Instead of heeding that cry, governments have shifted from housing strategies to homelessness strategies. Rather than planning how to get people into stable homes, we are looking at how to get them short-term shelter. Aside from not delivering what people really need, short-term shelter can cost five to ten times as much as long-term housing.[3] This after-the-fact approach is analogous to the spending on health care over disease prevention, where governments find themselves spending far more money to clean up messes rather than a reasonable amount preventing them. It's like a family that decides they should eat at restaurants because groceries cost too much. Doing the math shows that a lot more is saved by up-front expenditures; a bit of foresight can save a great deal of expense down the line. Our governments are increasingly reacting, not planning, renting, not owning, and, as a result, costing themselves out of all kinds of essential services. The decision of governments to live hand-to-mouth rather than plan ahead results in worse outcomes for more money. If our friends and neighbours acted that way, we'd shake our heads and think their priorities were confused. Why do we insist on this kind of behaviour from those who manage our taxes?

On a system level, public investment in affordable housing has many advantages. Job creation at various skill levels occurs near the communities with the highest unemployment. While there are initial investments required, before long public money is saved in health, justice, and social services. By shifting people from homeless to renting, from renting to owning, and from social assistance to employment, a comprehensive housing strategy can decrease costs and increase tax revenues. It can also present opportunities to use what we learn about planning and design to create safe, inclusive, sustainable communities.

Decreasing the percentage of monthly income spent on housing also helps to address food insecurity, the inability of people to reliably access the food they need to live healthy, active lives.[4] Two million Canadians experience food insecurity, and Aboriginal families like the Bouviers are three times as likely to find themselves in this situation as non-Aboriginals.[5] Nearly one million Canadians accessed food banks in 2010,[6] a number that has risen sharply in recent years. That same year, the number of people accessing food banks in booming Saskatchewan rose by twenty per cent.[7] While the people who run and volunteer at food banks do admirable work, they are limited in what they can provide. Charitable approaches can even pose an obstacle to addressing food insecurity,[8] serving as band-aid solutions for deeper problems. Programs are needed that address not only access to affordable food but also the poverty that makes that access difficult.

Some local initiatives offer hopeful examples, such as CHEP Good Food Inc.[9] Starting out as a school meal program, this nutrition-oriented, community-based organization now manages multiple community gardens and collective kitchens in Saskatoon's core neighbourhoods, helping people to produce and prepare healthy food. They also run the Good Food Box, a bulk buying and distribution program that makes fruit, vegetables, and grains, many purchased from local producers, available regularly at reduced prices. They are also the force behind the development of the Good Food Junction, the community-owned and operated grocery store intended to serve as a commercial anchor at Station 20 West. These programs are models of the ways in which an approach to food security needs to involve links between agriculture, food distribution systems, education, and economic development. By themselves, however, community based-organizations simply cannot meet the need. There is an important role here for corporate social responsibility, with commodity, wholesale, and retail food marketers needing to play their part in ensuring the services they offer are available to all people, even if profit margins are less than they might be in bigger cities and wealthier neighbourhoods.

The co-operative sector has also been instrumental in the past in addressing access to affordable food, and could be again. Where companies are unable or unwilling to provide services, there needs to be a co-ordinated effort from governments at all levels to make sure the proper incentives and regulations are in place to make good quality food accessible and affordable for everyone.

A Wider World

One way for us to get our house in order as a society is to address basic needs like food and shelter more equitably. We need a plan to ensure that people can afford safe places to live and good food to eat. An essential part of that plan has to be ensuring that the homes we build and the food we grow are safe for the world around them. Our homes are our most immediate connection with the external environment. Whether it's energy and resource use or waste production, polluting patterns of transportation or displacement of natural ecosystems, human habitation is a close-to-home example of the way human activity affects the larger environment.

No serious discussion of the way we view our society can ignore the growing concerns about our effects on the health of the ecosystems that support human life. Discourse on the determinants of health has tended to focus more on the impact of the immediate environments, while ignoring larger concepts of sustainable living. Though the focus on the immediate impacts of individual circumstances is important, it's also clear that air and water quality, climate change, and consumption of limited resources have significant effects on our health. We are creatures of our environment, and our health is greatly affected by the air we breathe, the plants and animals we eat, the water we drink, and our ability to live without fear of natural disasters.

The past two years in the prairie provinces of Alberta, Saskatchewan, and Manitoba have offered stark examples of the effects of climate change on local environments. Severe weather events and extreme temperatures are increasingly common. Forest fires and floods chase people from their homes. Simultaneous flooding and droughts threaten the safety and availability of potable water, and prevent farmers from seeding or harvesting crops. Over time, this instability can impede our ability to predict weather cycles for food production, and with that the ability of people to make a living in agriculture.

There may be no other industry so intimately linked with ecology as agriculture. The way in which we farm, be it through choices of transport methods, pest and weed control, or simply location and intensity, has huge implications for soil quality, erosion, climate change, and water safety. The role of the farmer as producer and steward of the land is one with enormous importance for the health of us all; policy decisions made through a health lens would necessarily involve helping producers to transition into methods that are both economically and environmentally sustainable. They would also explore macro level changes — around fossil fuel use, climate change, and commodity markets — that affect the environment in which farmers operate.

It's Hot in the Poor Places Tonight

While the frequency and intensity of environmental catastrophes have increased in recent years, in Canada they have tended to cause little direct harm to humans. That certainly has not been the case in other countries. As a young man I travelled to South America to learn what life was like in the developing world. I was hosted for the first few weeks in the Saskatoon Roman Catholic Diocese mission in União dos Palmares, in the North Eastern Brazilian state of Alagoas. Brazil is one of the world's most striking examples of income inequality, a land known for astoundingly wealthy gated communities overlooking sprawling slum cities, or *favelas*. What is seen locally in the large cities of the South plays out geographically as well, with the North East the poorest part of South America's economic giant. There the incomes and health status of most people are similar to Sub-Saharan Africa. With crumbling colonial Portuguese architecture and a large Afro-Brazilian population descended from the slave trade, the similarities between life in Brazil and Mozambique are striking.

The one major difference is industrial. While Mozambicans largely rely on subsistence farming, agriculture in Brazil is far more industrial. The North East is one of the world's largest providers of sugar. Almost all the agricultural land is used for this purpose, and a large percentage of the population works in factories or cutting cane. Much of the product goes to the Coca-Cola Company, which has significant interests in the area. A small number of *latifundários*, or large landowners, control the vast majority of land (in Brazil, one per cent of landowners own nearly half the arable land[10]), having over centuries forced most small farmers into feudal service in the cane fields. Fruit orchards and forests have been converted en masse to sugar cane, causing major changes in local ecosystems.

The town of União is located on the river Mundaú in the shadow of the famous Serra da Barriga (Belly Mountain). The Serra was the seat of government for Zumbi dos Palmares, the leader of a slave revolt that overthrew the Portuguese and ruled the region for nearly 100 years in the 17th century. Each year, pilgrims gather in the historic town, march across the bridge that spans the river, and make the long trek up the mountain in a celebration of resistance and a call for justice.

In May and June the rains are always heavy, but in 2010 they came heavier than usual. With almost all the land in the area deforested for cattle and cane, the water poured down out of the hills in torrents. The Mundaú had flooded before, and people in the streets by the river knew the risk, but it had never been like this. Entire towns in its path were demolished. Water crushed homes, churches, and hospitals. While some advance warning kept the immediate casualties down, a few dozen people were swept away, and many more were seriously injured, overwhelming what local health facilities were left standing. In the medium term, hundreds of families were left homeless, crowded into refugee camps plagued with water-borne illnesses and mini-epidemics of respiratory infections. A year later, many of the flood victims face an uncertain future: unable to return to rebuild where they were before, and unsure whether the flood relief donations will be enough for a new community to materialize. Disruption in schooling, food shortages, unstable housing, unemployment, and tragic family losses will affect the health of an entire generation.

This tragedy is compounded by the fact that it was completely avoidable. Organizations like Movimento Sem Terra (the landless farmers movement) have been advocating for land reform and sustainable farming practices in the region for decades. Successive governments have promised change, but the forces resisting agrarian reform are powerful. More responsible land use could have prevented, or at least minimized, the flooding. In a more equitable society, fewer people would have to live on the marginal riverbank land. And if flooding did happen, there would be more resilience in personal resources and social safety nets, as we see when similar events occur in Canada.

Canada is one of the world's largest contributors to greenhouse gases, with Saskatchewan the highest per capita contributor in the country.[11] There are aspects of our environment that contribute to this: cold winters and long distances to travel mean more energy use, fossil fuel intensive industries like mining, oil, and agriculture contribute to emissions. That may explain some of the unequal impact we are having on the environment, but it doesn't excuse it. We benefit greatly from the use of non-renewable resources, and the associated production of carbon and other pollutants. With the prosperity purchased through that production comes a responsibility to do things differently. The river metaphor comes to life in the Mundaú in Brazil, the Souris in Southern Saskatchewan, the raging Red in Manitoba. The downstream effects of climate change are detrimental to human health at home and abroad. Fortunately, Canada is also in a position (physically and fiscally, if not yet politically) to do something upstream. We have enormous resources in wind, sun, and geothermal energy. We are able to do some of the forward thinking and investing required to save resources and energy and decrease our impact on the wider environment. While investing in conservation and converting to renewable energy have up-front costs, the long-term savings in energy use make it a more than worthwhile investment. If we take action soon enough, there is potential for significant job creation in growth industries related to renewable energy. If a healthy population for generations to come is our goal, we would be foolish not to try to shift to practices that prevent damage to the eco-systems that support us.

Environmental impact is the most upstream of policy considerations, one that intersects with every other policy area. Balancing the various determinants requires moving beyond simple dichotomies of jobs and trees to making the complex and challenging decisions to ensure long-term environmental and economic sustainability. Human health can give us a guiding principle through which to make these choices, doing our best to enact the policies that create the conditions for optimal health.

Bringing it Home

Sometimes one person's story can remind us why we care about the bigger picture. Coming back to Jessica and Elaine, we see how the immediate environment is affecting her health. Talking to her mother, it was clear that, while she is trying to provide for her family, her housing situation is making it impossible to get ahead. Hoping to improve the situation, the social worker at West Side got her in touch with Quint Development Corporation, a local housing and community development organization. Along with running affordable housing units and transition homes for young men and women in need of housing support, Quint also runs a co-op housing program, helping families to go from renters to home owners. In building and renovating, they concentrate on energy efficiency to decrease the impact on the environment as well as decrease utility costs for members. Elaine and her family have established themselves in one of the apartment complexes, and are hoping to join the co-op program and eventually own their own house.

After a few months in their new Quint apartment, things have really settled down for Elaine and her children. Elaine got a job at a daycare and is making more than she took in on social assistance. A lower rent is taking less of the family income, allowing them to make better choices in groceries, and even afford some new school clothes for Jessica. She's been at the same school for the longest time since grade one, and while she still struggles, there has been some improvement. An educational assistant has been assigned to her and is helping her to catch up on some areas she'd missed in all the moves. She's still a handful, but she's made some friends and even says she likes her school. We decide to wait and see before trying any medication, hoping that the more stable home will continue to improve things for Jessica.

If we want children like Jessica to do better in their lives, we need to make sure they have more than the bare minimum to survive in the world. A decent income, stable housing, clean water, nutritious food, and good quality education are necessary elements of the home life required to thrive in the wider world.

There are many things that can be done to improve the circumstances of families like Jessica's. Programs like those offered by Quint are great, but their reach is limited. There is a need for programs of greater scope. Private companies cannot be expected to produce low-income housing on their own, but they can be encouraged to do so through tax incentives and percentage requirements of affordable units in any new developments. Accompanied by the purchase and construction of housing units by multiple levels of government, this can increase the available housing stock, and reduce or eliminate the waiting lists and the growing number of people who are homeless. This will also decrease costs, as money spent on housing will be saved in emergency shelters and rooms. This is, on a large-scale, the same sort of home economy we would teach young people and those in need: it is better to save than to borrow, to own than to rent, to maintain than to replace, to invest than to spend. These are important lessons, and when applied to policy decisions they make sense. What is needed is the political will to make them happen.

The key to mobilizing that political will is for people to recognize that the world around us, from massive eco-systems right down to our living rooms, has a great deal to do with the quality of our lives. With health as a well-articulated, overarching public goal, we can demand of our representatives that they take the necessary steps to make sure we become healthier and stay that way. That pressure, translated into public demand and votes, will enable leaders to preserve and improve the physical environments that support us.

CHAPTER 5

The Equality of Mercy

The opening of every schoolhouse closes a jail.

François Guizot

Down by Law

In my first year of practice, working at the West Side Community Clinic in Saskatoon, I met a young man whose story has come to represent for me the problems with the justice system. While normally I would change his name and some details to protect his privacy, Brad Peequaquat has been brave enough to share his story with the Saskatoon StarPhoenix.[1] When I first met Brad he had only recently had an extensive, disfiguring surgery to remove a cancer of the penis. This was radical treatment, necessary to save his life, at least temporarily, from a quickly spreading cancer. Had it been caught earlier he may not have needed such a surgery and the long-term hope of survival would have been much higher.

The problem is, it was caught earlier. Brad had been to see his family doctor when the cancer was a small but concerning lesion on his foreskin. He saw a urologist and an appointment was made for a circumcision, a benign and usually curative procedure if done early enough. Unfortunately, he never made the appointment.

Brad grew up in a family with a father who was violently abusive and who regularly committed break-ins and other property crimes. Shown little else in the way of options, Brad and his brothers followed suit, robbing liquor stores and bars and selling the proceeds in inner-city Saskatoon. This activity brought him to the attention of the Indian Posse, a gang based out of Winnipeg, and he became one of the local leaders in Saskatoon. Like most of the gang members, he was in and out of prison on various charges.

Unlike most of those young men, Brad had a change of heart. He met a woman he cared about, his wife Joanne, and decided to leave the gang life in favour of fatherhood. Helped by a Saskatoon organization called Str8Up, run by Catholic priest André Poilièvre, he and his brothers found the strength to leave the gang. Things were really turning around for Brad, but in 2007 he was caught drinking in violation of his parole and sentenced to a month in prison.

This is where things went really wrong. Brad showed the prison staff the letter about his appointment for surgery. Everything was arranged for him to be taken from jail to the hospital for the circumcision. However, it was a tense time in the corrections system, with a recent high-profile escape, and the guards appear to have been exercising more than their usual control over prisoners. Peequaquat phoned his surgeon's office to talk about his condition, an action in violation of prison policy.

In retribution, the prison staff chose not to give him an escort, and his surgery date came and went. By the time he was released and saw the surgeon again, the cancer had spread locally and to distant lymph nodes. A circumcision would no longer suffice; radical surgery was needed, causing significant disability and pain and little hope of long-term survival. In May 2011, Brad passed away, leaving behind his wife and a young family.

Brad's story is a monumental tragedy. It is also a glaring example of a justice system that is designed to punish rather than to prevent and protect. This is analogous to a medical system that is curative rather than preventive. The results are the same: more expense, less effect. The people who need help are met late in the progression of their illness, or their criminal behaviour, too late to make real change. How much easier, and more effective, is it to keep people from smoking than getting them to stop? How much wiser to keep people out of jail than to try to rehabilitate them once they're in.

Determining Detention

The same factors that determine one's health determine one's likelihood to come into contact with the justice system. If we look at the Canadian prison population, the inmates are overwhelmingly of lower social economic status, and have low levels of formal education.[2] They are also disproportionately Aboriginal, with twenty per cent of the prison population in Canada compared to three per cent of the general public. In Saskatchewan

Aboriginal people make up ten per cent of the overall population and an astonishing fifty-seven per cent of the prison population.[3] The same factors that lead to ill health — poverty, low levels of education, social exclusion, racial discrimination, unemployment — also lead to imprisonment.

If we want to improve health outcomes, we need to address the root causes of illness. Similarly, if we want to decrease crime, we need to address its root causes as well. What is fortunate is that they are the same things. While the justice system hasn't usually been described as one of the major factors in determining health (the numbers of people in prison are still small enough that it doesn't have the same statistical impact as the other factors to which all are exposed), it's clear that incarceration has a substantial impact on health status.

Another way of looking at this is to see it as a companion indicator of social health: the determinants of health are the determinants of involvement in criminal behaviour. Rising or falling crime rates are clear indicators of whether or not we have been successful in producing a safe society, not through intimidation and deterrence, but through an appropriate distribution of opportunity and the common wealth. This is important to consider when designing policy responses to try to make Canada a safer country: are more prisons and tougher sentences the right answer? It depends on what you're trying to achieve.

There are three potential reasons to punish someone. The first is retribution: looking to exact a repayment for damage done. The second is risk management: seeking to protect others from the actions of someone who does not respect the law. The third is rehabilitation: seeking to correct the behaviour and teach the offender a better way.

In our private lives, in our own homes and families, we discourage revenge as a motivator. Most of us can think back to hear a parent admonishing a fighting child, "I don't care who started it, you have to stop it." While it is very tempting to get back at someone who has hurt us, upon sober reflection it is easy to see the ways in which that perpetuates conflict and justifies aggression. Is it not odd, then, that our judicial system, thought to represent the balanced wisdom of the best legal minds, focuses almost entirely on punishment? There is very little in the way of crime prevention, and not nearly enough rehabilitation.

The degree of civilization in a society can be judged by entering its prisons.

— Fyodor Dostoevsky[4]

One shocking move away from rehabilitation was the closure, in 2009, of the farms connected to prisons in cities like Kingston, Ontario and Prince Albert, Saskatchewan.[5] These farms provided food for the prisons and taught skills to the inmates. While inmates might not be destined to farm once on the outside, the day-to-day skills of showing up, applying themselves to a task, and experiencing the satisfaction of a day's work are invaluable developments that can be applied to a return to normal life in society. Rather than give people psychological help, or train them in work skills applicable to the outside world, it often appears the current system would rather see them sit aimless in jail.

With this approach, inmates at best return to life in society exactly where they left off, having just paused for a few years to reflect. More likely, however, they return worse than they came in, either as a result of having lost ground by going to jail, having been physically and psychologically traumatized, or having gotten further involved in criminality in prison through drug and gang activity. Most convicts leave prison with little waiting for them on the outside: nowhere to stay, little prospect for employment, and minimal social support. Returning unskilled and undesirable to general society is a recipe for desperation. Add to this the environment in which the last years have been spent, in the company of other criminals, in a culture of gangs, drugs, and violence, and repeat offence becomes even more predictable. Hence, the common description of prisons as institutions not of correction but of higher education in criminality. To return to the analogy of health, one could even see criminal behaviour as a nosocomial infection (one you catch in a hospital): for the susceptible, nowhere is as dangerous to your full recovery as an institution of the unwell like a hospital or a prison.

Incarceration rates are fed by the popular belief . . . that punishment reduces crime, a belief seemingly immune to evidence.

— David Cayley [6]

This makes the current emphasis in Canada on increased sentences and the expansion of prisons all the more disturbing. It reflects a further abandonment of prevention and a pursuit of an approach to crime akin to that of the United States. In the US, prison populations have skyrocketed in recent decades, with over two million people currently behind bars.[7] This has occurred despite an overall decrease in crime rates, largely as a result of increased harshness in sentencing and a focus on imprisonment over other forms of punishment. Given the large body of evidence of the failure of this approach, it's an example of ideologically driven decision-making trumping evidence-based policy. It also reflects a trend in Canada toward a less equal society, as Richard Wilkinson points out in *The Spirit Level*: "There is a strong social gradient in imprisonment, with people of lower class, income and education much more likely to be sent to prison than people higher up the social scale."[8] Corrections policies that emphasize imprisonment reflect a growing inequality and a growing tendency to view those of lower socio-economic status as dangerous, undeserving, and worthy of incarceration. The imprisonment of large numbers of marginalized people further marginalizes them, increasing the degree of social inequality.

Clearly, there is a problem here. The question is what to do about it. The big picture answer is the theme of this book: work to create a healthy society, a more equal society, a fairer society, and you will have a safer society by extension.

This won't happen overnight, however, and it won't mediate the damage done by the current justice system. To alleviate the negative impact of the ill-named correction system, there need to be significant reforms in our approach to crime.

Safety in Numbers — The Evidence for Clemency

An effective justice system must measure its success mainly on how well it can change harmful behaviour into socially useful behaviour. We must reduce those techniques which have the side effect of increasing crime. These techniques (incarceration being the most obvious example) are expensive. It costs anywhere from $50,000 to over $150,000 a year to house a criminal in prison — depending on the level of security, whether it is a provincial or federal institution, or whether the convict is male or female.[9] With just under 40,000 prisoners in Canada on any given day, that's at least $2 billion per year (including parole and other non-inmate custody services, Canadians paid $3.9 billion in correctional costs in the 2008-2009 fiscal year).[10] How many at-risk youth could be helped and kept from offending with even a portion of that amount? Money saved through reform could be used to fund those organizations that have shown they are able to help people with multiple disadvantages from winding up in further trouble with the law.

Canada needs a criminal justice system that is effective. Such a system would (step 1) efficiently and accurately identify those who harm other citizens, and (step 2) use the most effective techniques for reducing the possibility that they may again harm other citizens. Our present methods do not focus on effective measures (step 2); instead, we focus on incarceration to attempt to "frighten" potential offenders. That technique has been proven to be worse than useless.

To understand why, we need to examine the possibility that a person, after release, will commit another offence (recidivism). The 2002 Public Safety Canada report, "The Effects of Punishment on Recidivism"[11] analyzed 111 separate, peer-reviewed studies which, in turn, studied over 400,000 offenders. The question was, once all variables were removed (i.e., sex, age, race), what is the difference when similar individuals were sentenced to prison terms or were placed on probation and allowed to live at home? The clear answer was that the incarcerated person was three to seven per cent more likely to commit another offence after release than a similar person who remained at home and was dealt with in the community. The seven per cent higher rate of recidivism relates to longer terms of incarceration.

There are many reasons for sending people to prison, but the conclusion that we should not rely on incarceration to reduce future crime is inescapable. Incarceration does not decrease crime. It increases it, and thus makes us less safe.

This dangerous side effect helps explain why democratic, wealthy countries with many similarities have different rates of incarceration which correspond to different crime rates. For example, the United States incarcerates several times more people per capita than do Canada, Germany, and Japan,[12] and also has a several times greater rate of murder and other serious crimes per capita than these same countries.[13] My home province of Saskatchewan, meanwhile, incarcerates more youth per capita than almost all other democratic, wealthy nations. We are moving toward disaster.

The majority of Canadian spending on reducing future harms goes to incarceration. If there are more effective techniques for decreasing crime, then doesn't it make more sense to reduce money spent on a technique that increases crime, such as incarceration, and use that same money on crime reduction techniques?

To further explore the impacts of determinants of health on involvement in the justice system, and exactly how just that system is, it is useful to ask, who goes to jail? If we look at incarcerated youth in Saskatchewan, they tend to be different from youth who are never incarcerated.

The most obvious difference is the number and seriousness of the problems the incarcerated youth inherit. They are far behind their peers in school; by the age of twelve or thirteen, almost all are roughly one to three years behind students of the same age.[14] Functional illiteracy is common, as it is in adult jails. Eighty per cent of them have a disability — some of them less serious learning disabilities, others more profound such as ADHD and Fetal Alcohol Spectrum disorders.[15] Ninety per cent come from families living in poverty.[16] Over eighty per cent are of a minority race, the vast majority Aboriginal.[17] More than half have had social services as their parent for at least some of their lives.[18] This latter statistic is particularly problematic; rather than helping parents in trouble keep their children, we take them away to foster care. Then, rather than help those children — damaged by the experience of separation from their families and often by the experience of life in foster care — stay out of trouble, we imprison them. This reactive response perpetuates the damage to families, particularly Aboriginal families damaged over generations through the reserve system, residential schools, and prolonged poverty, ensuring future generations of apprehended and incarcerated children. Assembly of First Nations national chief Shawn Atleo recently made headlines by stating that children growing up on reserves are more likely to go to prison than finish high school,[19] a statistic that can only be seen as a stain on the nation's reputation. Clearly, something must be done to turn this situation around.

Research, especially from health, education, and youth-oriented community groups, shows that more can be done, that we can work with these young people. Indeed, since groups such as Str8Up have as one of their goals encouraging youth to achieve their potential, they tend to transform these youth into successful citizens. Saskatchewan is fortunate to have many examples of successful programs, ranging from art education to conflict resolution, from employment education to canoeing with cops, from money management to drama. The more young people can be shown the process that leads from disadvantage to success, and just how enjoyable the process can be, the less likely they are to commit crimes. Unfortunately, most such organizations are starved for funds — living grant-to-mouth, as it were — and so their impact is not as great as it might be.

An effective justice system must measure its success mainly on how well it changes harmful behaviour to social usefulness (step 2). To do that, we must reduce those practices which have the side effect of increasing crime. The money saved should be used to fund organizations that have shown they can be successful at helping youth with multiple disadvantages not only to survive but to thrive. It can also be used to increase the focus in prison on rehabilitation. Building in intensive counselling and skills training, and creating privilege and sentence-related incentives that promote success in rehabilitation can make prisons into actual corrections facilities that prepare prisoners for a better, more responsible life on the outside rather than perpetuating criminal culture.

If we want a safer society, we need to aim for effective measures that really reduce crime and rely less on trying to frighten the marginalized. We need to use the evidence available to transform our justice system into a force for good. Again we see the parallel with health care, where what we currently have are revolving-door clinics, seeing people when they are ill, dealing with symptoms, but failing to address the reasons they become ill in the first place. This guarantees that they'll be back and sick again, just as a justice system that treats the symptom of crime with the medication of prison and fails to address the root causes of criminal behaviour ensures that we will have revolving-door prisons. Some suggest that this means we should mete out longer and tougher sentences; however, as the evidence shows, this only exacerbates the problem and increases repeat crime and incarceration. How much wiser would it be to work with people to get them out of the justice system than to keep them in as long as possible?

> "We need to get tough on poverty, poor housing, racism — the social issues that lead us down the road to crime."
> — Saskatoon Chief of Police Clive Weighill[20]

Coming back to Brad Peequaquat, I am struck by the enormous waste of opportunity. Here was a young man who tried to turn his life around. He sought help, but the system was only able to respond with negligence, enforcing the rules blindly. The result has been great financial cost for both the hospital and the justice system, the tragedy of pain, disability, and ultimately death for Brad, and great sadness for his family. For all of us, it means the loss of a bright young man who, given the opportunity, could have helped others to see that there were better choices than street life.

The implications of the parallels between justice and health are profound. The same issues that cause one to be ill — poverty, unemployment, poor education, nutrition, or housing — are those that predict one's likelihood of incarceration. It stands to reason that, if we invest in people's health and wellbeing, we will also be investing in crime prevention and the safety of all citizens. Finding creative ways to keep people out of the justice system and keep our streets safe at the same time are key to building a healthy society.

CHAPTER 6

Learning to Live

IN THE NEIGHBOURHOOD WHERE I WORK there are a lot of women who live in difficult circumstances. Some come in regularly to the clinic, seeing it as a safe place where people want to help. Others seek out different organizations like EGadz Street Outreach, AIDS Saskatoon, or Quint Housing Corporation. Others don't, or can't, or won't seek help at all. Amy is one of the latter, a twenty-six-year-old mother of three who hasn't been doing well. She's on social assistance, in an abusive relationship, and addicted to alcohol. Whether it's the strength of her addiction, her controlling partner, or just lack of belief that anyone will help her, she's been reluctant to get help. I see her occasionally in the clinic for acute issues, but she doesn't stay engaged or keep follow-up appointments, and she refuses offers of help to get out of her current situation. People like Amy can be frustrating, because there are ways to help them but they aren't ready to change, and there's little we can do to move them toward readiness.

In the past couple of months, however, I've been seeing a bit more of Amy and a bit more willingness to consider a new life. This isn't because of anything we've done at the clinic, it's due to her cousin, Mason. Mason works as an engineer, is politically and socially active, and in general a pretty together young man. When you hear the stories of his family of origin, it's clear just how unlikely an outcome this was. Alcohol, drugs, poverty, and petty crime were around him all the time growing up. His father died from the complications of a lifelong alcohol addiction. Many of his relatives are in prison, or imprisoned by poverty and addictions. The question that stories like Mason's always bring to mind is, why did he bounce when those around him fell flat? Why is he succeeding when so many of his cousins, peers, and friends have ended up in situations as bad or worse than the generation before them? He's a healthy young man enjoying a good life, but many of the determinants of health in his upbringing — income, social status, physical environment — worked against that. Why was he able to take the hardships and use them as reasons to succeed rather than excuses not to?

Mason attributes it to the fact that, when things got really bad with his parents, he went to stay with his maternal grandfather, a math and history teacher. Life at his grandfather's was different: there was enough to eat, they weren't constantly moving, and no one was drunk. In these more peaceful times, Mason's grandfather taught him how to learn and helped him develop a talent for math. Math became his escape when things got bad, and eventually the balloon that lifted him up where no one thought he'd go.

While school was a struggle for him socially — he was often excluded because of his race and status — he could count on getting decent marks. At university he found a more welcoming social scene and thrived in the College of Engineering. Now, along with a successful job as an engineer, he works with young people in Saskatoon's inner city, tutoring math and helping others find the talent that will help them out of poverty and despair.

Mason is a remarkable individual, but according to him one thing is clear: school helped. He was fortunate enough to live in a place where there was no distinction between the good school and the bad school. There was just school. And he had talented teachers, including his grandfather, who recognized his potential and challenged him along the way. When he struggled, he got extra help; when he was bored, he was challenged.

Education is recognized as one of the key determinants of health. The higher the level of education an individual can achieve, the more likely they are to live a long and healthy life. Like income, education also has an impact on the other determinants. Level of education is strongly correlated with income, as those with more training and skills can command higher levels of pay, as well as better employment opportunities and working environments. The literacy and numeracy skills obtained through education affect the way people access housing and health care, and the choices they make around nutrition, physical activity, smoking, and substance use. Social skills obtained during schooling contribute to the formation of social support networks.

The process of education, both curricular and informal, is in general one that contributes to a healthy life. Where there is a common public school system, accessible to all, education is a force for greater equality in society.

Education then, beyond all other devices of human origin, is the great equalizer of the conditions of men, the balance-wheel of the social machinery.

— Horace Mann[1]

A Class Apart

The degree to which education is effective in its role as equalizer is dependent on the same elements as health care: access, quality, and affordability. While in most of Canada we are still fortunate enough to have good public schools, gaps in access and quality are cause for concern. There are inequities between rural and urban schools at all levels, as well as differences in quality of education and extra-curricular opportunities depending on community incomes.

One example of a growing gap is that of schools on First Nations reserves. In the fall of 2011, the Cree First Nation of Attawapiskat declared a state of emergency that brought national attention, including a fundraising campaign through the Canadian Red Cross. Housing had deteriorated in quality and availability, with many of the 1500 band members living in poorly built, overcrowded shelters without indoor plumbing and without adequate insulation and heating to withstand a northern Ontario winter. The current housing crisis is only the latest in a long list of troubles for Attawapiskat, including insufficient water treatment facilities and pollution from a large diesel spill under the elementary school. The diesel spill led to health problems among children and teachers, and the school was demolished, as it should have been. What didn't follow was a new school. Successive federal governments have refused to build a replacement, leading community youth to start a campaign which has become known as Shannen's Dream,[2] after Shannen Koostachin, a student champion who, prior to her death in a car accident at age fifteen, was nominated for the International Children's Peace Prize as a representative of the children who advocated for a new school.

What other Canadian kid has to fight, organize and beg for access to clean and equitable schools?

— Charlie Angus, MP
Timmins-James Bay, Ontario[3]

The story of Attawapiskat is a particularly strong example of the inequality of experience and opportunity faced by First Nations children. Indian and Northern Affairs Canada, by placing a two per cent per year growth cap on education spending in a time of population growth, has legislated long-term underfunding.[4] On average, on-reserve schools are funded a third less per student than schools in the rest of Canada — all of this when Aboriginal students have the highest educational needs, including the lowest level of completion of secondary education, and schools that are described as being two grades behind those of comparable schools off reserve.

This inattention and underfunding doesn't make a lot of sense. What teacher, presented with a student who was struggling in school, would intentionally give them a third less attention than the other students? Students in difficulty receive more attention, and rightly so. Wise teachers know that the earlier they address the difficulties of a struggling student, the brighter the future for that student and the better the experience for the entire class. The same wisdom should be applied to addressing key determinants of health such as education among the communities most in need, be they urban, rural or on-reserve; greater attention and resources should be applied to deal with greater challenges.

The Education Advantage

The challenges in education don't end at grade 12. When entering the work force, young people face increased post-secondary education requirements, but greater impediments to their pursuit. Tuition has risen dramatically at universities across the country. Adding to that higher costs of living, particularly for students who need to leave home to attend school, potential students from low-income families are choosing not to seek further training. Those who do face debt burdens on graduation that serve as obstacles to further study or becoming established in their careers and businesses. Student loan debt reduction has been falling, with provincial governments moving toward tax rebates for graduates. While this is appealing for governments, as they don't increase expenditures and potentially can have some impact on the recruitment of graduates to stay in the province, it does nothing to reduce the upfront costs faced by students.

One striking change, which typifies the current direction but has gone largely without debate, is the practice of differential tuition for professional schools like Medicine and Law. The idea that, since they will eventually earn more, students in these colleges should pay higher tuition (often two to three times that of students in other colleges), makes sense on the surface. However, when considered more deeply, it becomes clear that this will exclude people from lower income and non-urban families. This results in a system where education acts not as an equalizing force in society, but something that preserves social difference. The result is not only less opportunity for those with greater needs, but also a less representative workforce in important fields of service.

An educated, healthy populace is our goal. It's also a positive feedback loop, an economic driver in itself. Removing barriers of access allows people to live fuller lives. It is also an investment in future prosperity, as healthy, educated people are better able to contribute to a society that produces healthy, educated people.

Canada has historically been a leader in public education investment, with affordable, quality institutions at all levels. However, during the budget crises of the 1990s, public investment was significantly cut and has never recovered to previous per-capita levels.[5] This has affected access through rising tuition costs; it has also affected quality, with increased class sizes and reducing or eliminating key areas of study. Not only is this failure to invest in education unwise for the health of the population, it's also a strategic error economically. It is a backward step to tie ourselves to an economy based solely on natural resources. Rather than being leaders in the emerging knowledge economy, we leave ourselves vulnerable to changes in commodity and labour markets. Investing in quality education will develop a generation with the skills not only to adapt to economic and technological advances but also to lead the way in their development.

Learning to Learn

[Education] is, or should be, concerned with changing the motivation that determines the direction of our seeking and moving so that society can be built on a firm foundation of human values. . . . Education should result not just in better trained hands and minds, but also in greater hearts.

— Woodrow Lloyd[6]

It is not enough to prepare learners for the workforce of today; we need to give them the skills to think critically and adapt to change in a world that may bear little resemblance to the one in which we currently live. Education is about more than simply obtaining the skills to succeed financially and live comfortably. There are facts to learn, of course, key concepts and information to digest and understand. More important, however, is learning literacy, the ability to apply critical thinking and skills in knowledge acquisition to adapt to a changing world. This requires literacy in household management, personal development, environmental stewardship, and in how to find and create employment.

It also applies directly to making choices in personal health. An important element of making wise choices is health literacy, the ability to access, understand, and act on information for health. This ranges from simple things like understanding immunizations or medications to making wise decisions in diet, exercise, and addictions, and being able to manage psychologically difficult periods of life, turning the anxiety and depression of tumultuous times into opportunities for personal growth.

People who have higher levels of education are more likely, on average, to get stable, well-paying jobs or to be successful in business. More and more jobs require higher levels of education. These facts cause confusion, as people conflate the results with the underlying purpose. People start to think that, because education leads to employment and material success, that's what education is for. As human beings, we are far more than our jobs and our bank accounts, and the goals of our learning must reflect a deeper sense of purpose.

Perhaps the greatest goal of education is not a set of skills, but the development of values. Our democracy is only as healthy as the next generation of youth and their ability to engage creatively with the world around them. Civic literacy means teaching youth not to be future subjects, observers of the news, but actors in the lives of their communities.

One of the best ways for governments to perpetuate the ability to make bad decisions for the majority, with the support of the majority, is to diminish the quality of education. Some educational theorists, such as the University of Ottawa's Dr. Joel Westheimer, have suggested that this is one motivation for education reforms in the United States, and some parts of Canada, that emphasize standardized testing on defined facts and skills, decreasing the amount of time available for civic education and critical thinking.[7] School curricula in previous decades allowed space for the discussion of social and environmental concerns, often acting as the fuel for student activism. This sort of content should be encouraged, as it can lead to young people who are more engaged with the world around them. It can lead them to participate more fully in democracy, and even to lead the kind of societal change that reflects the values taught in elementary school. Currently there is a disconnect between what is taught and the values exhibited by people in positions of authority.

In order to provide this kind of learning environment, we need first to value those who do the front line work. As I was writing this chapter, Saskatchewan's teachers had taken strike action for the first time in nearly eighty years. Like most strikes, the headlines come down to wages and percentages; the teachers wanting more, the government offering less, and the public in the middle wondering what's fair. As with most strikes, there were deeper questions that didn't make the headlines.

How do we value the work teachers do? If we are committed to the best education for young people, what is needed to make that happen? Clearly, it includes attracting bright, committed people to the teaching profession. This means not only paying them well, but also creating the kind of environment in which they and their students can thrive. To be effective at responding to and leading educational innovation, teachers need the opportunities to improve on their existing skills and learn additional and emerging techniques throughout their careers. Rather than going backward to a more prescriptive and less responsive system of education, or playing hard ball with teachers over their demands, we need to explore ways to advance the cause of learning at all levels.

Off to a Good Start

Early childhood experiences are key determinants of the health of children and the adults they will become. The biggest impact on these experiences is material privation; the approximately fifteen per cent of Canadian children living in poverty face an uphill climb when seeking healthy lives.[8] The interventions with the biggest impact on childhood health will be economic: lifting families with children out of poverty. Dr. Paul Kershaw, economist at the University of British Colombia, describes the current generation that is raising children as "generation squeezed," as they face increasing costs of living without associated increase in wages. For example, housing costs across Canada increased by seventy six per cent between 1976 and 2006, while household incomes only increased by six per cent in that period, despite there being nearly twice as many women in the workforce contributing to that household income.[9]

> The generation raising kids today is squeezed for time at home; they are squeezed for income because of the cost of housing, even when not "poor"; and they are squeezed for services like child care that will help them balance successfully raising a family with earning a living.
> — Paul Kershaw[10]

Aside from economic changes, there is an important role for the educational system as well. It goes beyond custodial day care to the goal of providing quality early educational experiences that help children develop the cognitive, language, and emotional skills to succeed in later life.

In Saskatchewan, we are nowhere near meeting this goal. The province has the lowest rate of child-care availability in the country, with less than ten per cent of children under six being accommodated.[11] Aside from being inconvenient for single-parent families, or families where both parents work, this child-care deficit decreases opportunities for implementing structured early childhood learning, and affects the provincial economy. In Quebec, where the provincial government has made child care available at $7 per day, the subsidy increases the number of women in the work force, and contributes to tax revenue by $1.50 for each dollar invested.[12] This is another of these remarkable instances where investment in human infrastructure pays for itself in the short term, without even considering the long-term benefits to the children and their families, which of course will be of long-term benefit to society as well in terms of increased productivity and decreased social cost. Expanding the opportunities for early childhood education, from enhanced child care to all-day kindergarten, is a cost-effective and evidence-based means of improving public health.

One of the more interesting means of making these changes is the concept of community schools, or "School Plus."[13] Community schools provide a focal point for neighbourhood services such as community associations, adult learning centres, paediatricians, nurses, psychologists, social workers, elders, addiction counsellors, and others. In the northern community of Île-à-la-Crosse there is a particularly shining example of this model. A bright yellow building, designed to resemble a sunset, looks out over the lake toward the historic island for which the town is named. This unique facility is anchored by two main tenants: St Joseph's Hospital and

Rossignol High School. St Joseph's is an acute care hospital with an emergency room, labs, an x-ray, and a long-term care centre. Rossignol High School has classroom, lab, and physical education facilities for students from Grade 7-12. In addition to the hospital and high school, there are a family medicine clinic, mental health counsellors, public health offices, and a community-run child care and early learning centre. With a library and gymnasium, a performing arts stage, meeting rooms and adult education classrooms, the Île-à-la-Crosse Integrated Services Centre is a one-stop-shop approach to addressing the determinants of health that expands the role of the school into a resource for everyone in the community, from newborns to elders.

While building new schools and hospitals is rarely an option, another appealing model is the integration of key services into existing facilities. St Mary's School in the inner-city Saskatoon neighbourhood of Pleasant Hill is host to a number of outreach initiatives from the local health region designed to address health inequities. These include an agility training program to address childhood obesity and inactivity, a nursing residency program that places nursing students in the classroom to work with children, and a paediatric clinic that offers clinical services in the school three days a week. By bringing the services to where the children are, rather than making families with limited means and multiple challenges come to appointments in other neighbourhoods, more kids get the help they need.

Higher Education

To free ourselves from the boom-and-bust cycle of principally resource-based economies, we need to ready ourselves for the knowledge economy of the future. Investment in K-12 education must be coupled with investment in post-secondary education, including professional colleges and technical schools, as well as basic sciences and humanities.

Poverty has always been a barrier to post-secondary education. With increasing tuition and related fees, a lack of affordable housing and the rising cost of nutritious food, post-secondary education is increasingly a challenge for young people from middle class and working families. Many choose not to seek higher education. Those who do often graduate with a burden of debt that will take them most of their working lives to pay off.

Education must be affordable and accessible for every young Canadian. While tax credits may be a useful means of keeping graduates in regions where they are needed, they are of little use if the cost of education keeps people out of school in the first place. Lowering barriers to post-secondary training, like subsidizing early childhood education, is an investment that pays off quickly in productivity and tax revenue and should be a priority for provincial and federal governments. This can be done by reducing tuition rates, increasing the number and amount of scholarships, targeting under-represented populations, simplifying and forgiving more student loans, and providing support to students who need to move to larger centres to continue their education. Taking affordable, practical steps to make education more accessible will allow us to prepare coming generations to lead us in advancing the health and wellbeing of all people.

A couple of weeks ago Amy came into the clinic and surprised me. She needed some lab work for another appointment, but had no real concerns. She'd moved into a new apartment and hadn't had a drink for over a month. Her partner is enrolled in anger management classes and she's looking at going back to school. While this change is her own success, she does attribute some of it to Mason's influence. By taking her kids for breaks, connecting Amy to the clinic, and just staying present in his cousin's life, he showed her there is a different way to live. The success of one family member through education was a bridge to a better life, evidence that there are smarter and healthier ways to live.

CHAPTER 7

Heading Downstream

By addressing the Social Determinants of Health you can provide better care and save money.
Canadian Medical Association president Jeff Turnbull[1]

Early in my medical career I spent a few years working as what is called a *locum tenens*, Latin for place-holder. Essentially I was a bookmark in the practice stories of other physicians, giving them a break and making sure that the people they work for could still see a doctor. This was an exciting job. It introduced me to new towns, new people, and new ways of practicing medicine. With a fascinating mix of emergency, clinic, and long-term care, in facilities new to me, it also kept me on my toes.

Of the many challenging situations, there is one that sticks out for me in particular. The day after Boxing Day in 2008, I was staying in a small town west of Saskatoon. At around 10:30, a lady named Lynn Peters who was experiencing chest pain and difficulty breathing came into the emergency room. She'd had the same thing before and had wound up in hospital, but wasn't sure what the cause had been.

Her legs were swollen. I listened to her lungs. They sounded a little bit wet, probably mild pulmonary edema. Those two together often mean heart failure. An ECG, an electrical tracing of her heart, showed the classic "tombstone" shape that indicates a myocardial infarction: a heart attack. I talked to the cardiologist on call in Saskatoon, and faxed her the ECG to double check. She agreed it looked like a heart attack and we decided, given the distance to Saskatoon, to try TNK. Heart attacks are caused by blood clots in the arteries that feed the heart. When they're plugged, the heart muscle starts to die. TNK is a clot-buster, breaking down the clot to open up blood flow to the heart. Done in time, this essentially reverses the heart attack and helps prevent serious damage. I'd never used it before, so the cardiologist reviewed the steps with me and then I did what happens so often in the field. I tried something I'd only read about.

This time, it failed. Whether as a result of or despite the TNK, suddenly her breathing got worse. Far worse. Her lungs now sounded like they were underwater, and there was pink foam coming from her mouth. Her blood oxygen levels had dropped from ninety-eight per cent to sixty per cent, despite having an oxygen mask on at full flow. I would have to put a tube in to help her breathe.

This I'd done before, but not since residency, not in this hospital, and never without a more experienced doctor present. Once again I chose to phone a friend. Despite the late hour, I called one of my classmates, an emergency physician who does intubations all the time. I told him my plan. He gave me some tips on how much of which medicine to use to paralyze her muscles and make her unconscious while the nurses adjusted her position and got the equipment ready. Whether it was my inexperience or just a very tough patient (the tissues of her tongue and throat were extremely swollen), I couldn't get her tubed, not even with special instruments, and neither could the ambulance staff. At one point her oxygen levels dropped into the forties and I found myself running around the unfamiliar emergency room looking for a scalpel to cut into her trachea and make an emergency airway.

Fortunately, I managed to insert a laryngeal mask airway (a rescue breathing device that works nearly as well as an endotracheal tube) and get her oxygen saturation back up to ninety per cent with a bag-valve mask, squeezing each breath into her lungs. And we kept doing so the whole way to Saskatoon. At -35°C, two nurses and I moved her into the back of the ambulance and took turns breathing for her for two and a half hours as the ambulance sped down the pot-holed highway to Saskatoon. Miraculously, we managed to keep the LMA in place, despite the bumps, and keep Lynn clinically stable until we arrived at the Royal University Hospital, where the emergency team took over, the anaesthesiologist intubated her, and the cardiologists went to work to see what could be done for her heart and lungs.

A couple of days later I was finished my service in that town and came back to Saskatoon. I went to the hospital to see how Mrs. Peters was doing. When I walked into her room, she was sitting up in bed having lunch. Her breathing was fine. I had to introduce myself because she didn't remember anything of what had happened that night. All she knew is that she came in to the hospital feeling sick, and now she was in Saskatoon feeling good, anxious to be discharged home.

This is an example of the most exciting and thrilling part of health care: using the skills of the health care team and the resources of the system to save people from the brink of death. Even for the trained and practiced, it's scary as hell. Avoiding emergencies, and all the times when people aren't as lucky as Lynn, is in many ways the point of this book. Her story, however, illustrates the importance of downstream care as one element of ensuring a healthy population.

As I mentioned earlier, health services fall further down the list of the determinants of health, and much of this book is about the changes that need to be made politically to avoid health problems. It is estimated that non-health care determinants account for three quarters of health outcomes. However, the other quarter is important, and downstream responses still have an important role to play in addressing quality of life. As well as being a safety net for when prevention and primary care fail, health care is a useful means of knowing about that failure. The number of people accessing emergency rooms, getting diagnosed with major illnesses, or needing surgery, are an accurate measure of whether we have been doing the upstream work to achieve healthier populations.

Of course, the measurement has to be done carefully. Like GDP growth, general improvements in health outcomes can be misleading, masking deep inequalities. While the overall trend in Canada is toward increases in life expectancy, in many parts of the country those at the bottom of the socio-economic scale are sicker and dying sooner. Public health research needs to be thorough and creative in order to use illness statistics to draw a clear picture of Canadian health.

One of the ways of ensuring that the right treatment is available for those who are ill is to make sure we have a health care system that is, as described in the *Canada Health Act*, universal, comprehensive, accessible, portable, and publicly administered. Designing services, from immunization programs to surgical wards, that meet the priority health concerns of those most in need, can contribute significantly to improvements in health status.

To begin, we must first recognize a couple of things about the current system. One is the great strides that have been made. The introduction of Medicare, a universal health insurance program for all Canadians, is one of the most remarkable accomplishments of our nation. It has resulted in better and fairer provision of health services, as well as a better understanding of the health problems faced throughout the country. The second is to acknowledge that the system is not perfect. There are inefficiencies in access and delivery, and barriers to change that make it costlier and less effective than it could be.

Care Where and When It's Needed

Not long ago, my wife Mahli was doing an elective in adolescent medicine in Toronto as part of her residency in paediatrics. She was five months pregnant and feeling unwell enough that she needed to see a doctor. While we were reluctant to go to the hospital in a strange city, we decided we needed to be sure that everything was all right. We went to the famous Mount Sinai hospital, walked into emergency and were sent straight up to the obstetrics floor. We were well-treated, all the appropriate tests were done, and in two hours we were heading home again, reassured. At no time were we told that we weren't welcome because we were from another province, asked about our ability to pay, or made to feel as though we were wasting time and money. We were amazed at the quality of care and ease of access.

In stark contrast is an experience from a few years ago. I was visiting friends on a reserve in northern Saskatchewan. It was mid-February and about -20°C, and I decided to go for a cross-country ski out on the lake. After about half an hour a man drove up to me on a snowmobile.

"Are you the doctor?" he asked.

I said yes, assuming he recognized me from previous visits and just wanted to say hi.

"Get on, there's been an accident."

We sped into town to the clinic, which is staffed by two very capable registered nurses and has a weekly "doctor day" when a doc from a nearby town flies in to see any patients the nurses are concerned about.

There we found Brandon, a teenage boy who'd been in a traffic accident. He'd been the passenger on a quad, a four-wheel all-terrain vehicle, that had slid into the back of a truck at the only stop sign in town. He was thrown from the quad into the path of an oncoming truck and run over. On examination, he was barely conscious, had two broken legs and a pretty serious head injury. I worked with the nurses and a medical student who was there visiting with me, to prepare him for transport. As a team, we splinted his legs, stabilized his neck, started lines, and got him into an ambulance. The ambulance sped down a gravel road to a town an hour away, from where he was flown another hour to Saskatoon for surgery and weeks of rehabilitation. As a team, we'd turned Brandon's very bad luck slightly better, making a potentially fatal accident into something he'll recover from in time.

Like most doctors, I have a collection of this kind of story, of being in the right place at the right time, and being made painfully aware of how often the opposite must be true. It was pure chance that we were there to help Brandon, and there are stories from across the country, in small towns, inner-city neighbourhoods, and on reserves, where people aren't as lucky, where access to health care is neither timely nor reliable. The recruitment of trained professionals is difficult, and many who are recruited come for brief periods, don't understand local issues, and may actually impede the delivery of quality care. For health services to have the impact they should in determining health, they have to be delivered when and where they're needed. Unfortunately, that is not the case for the poorest third of Canadians.[2]

Responding to the Needs of Society

Saskatchewan's medical school is well aware of these issues and has for the past several years been host to an active Social Accountability Committee. Social accountability, as defined by the World Health Organization, is the obligation of medical schools to "meet the priority health needs of the communities they serve."[3] This group looks to identify unmet health needs in Saskatchewan and beyond and to direct the activities of the college in Clinical activity, Advocacy, Research, Education and training (known as the CARE model)[4] to address these needs. This work has resulted in, among other things, the creation of some innovative programs to teach medical students about service.

One program that exposes students to real life situations with the intention of giving them a deeper understanding of the determinants of health is called Making the Links. Students in this program spend time volunteering at SWITCH, the student-run clinic in inner-city Saskatoon. They also work in communities in Northern Saskatchewan, including the reserve where Brandon was injured. In the final phase of the program, these same students work in a hospital in the small town of Massinga, in Mozambique. Through these varied experiences, with rural and remote Aboriginal communities, in an underserved urban setting, and in Sub-Saharan Africa, the students become intimately familiar with the ways in which social determinants affect people's health. By participating in this community service-learning, contributing to the local communities while learning about the health issues they face, students move beyond learning dry concepts in a classroom setting to real connections with people and their stories. The relationships they form are personal and meaningful and lead them to a deeper understanding of patients as people and of the factors in their lives that determine whether or not they'll be healthy.

While the effects of this program on individual students are huge, its scope is small. If we are really going to see that health care services are offered where and how they're needed, it will require substantial changes. Some of these will be in training, with more physicians, nurses, and other health care professionals being trained in the communities most in need of service. That will lead to greater understanding of rural or inner-city life, the development of relationships with and affinity for communities, and lead more people to choose to serve where they are needed.

Change in the way health care is provided, and paid for, also needs to happen. The primary way that physicians are paid is fee-for-service, with each patient visit being charged to the government based on the service rendered. This results in some perverse incentives away from the best quality care. For example, in Saskatchewan a clinic visit is classified as a 5B, and pays the same amount whether it's a cold or a new diagnosis of cancer. As you can imagine, these take very different amounts of time, knowledge, and concentration. In essence, the system encourages speedy care to minor problems and the avoidance of complexity. Shifting to salary or mixed payment schedules encourages physicians to spend more time at the front end of care, taking the time to address all the issues of a patient before they get out of hand. This is also a means of addressing the major discrepancy between the pay of specialists and the family doctors on the front line.

Reform in the way physicians, nurses, pharmacists, physiotherapists, and others work together can also make a big difference. By working together, primary health care teams can offer a holistic approach to patient care. This means more co-ordinated care, wiser use of the skills of highly trained professionals, and more attention to patient experience and what's really needed to make a difference in their lives.

As Sustainable as We Want it to Be

As a result of public administration, the cost of doctor and hospital services is relatively stable. Each has fallen as a portion of the total spending on health (private and public) in the country. So why are health costs taking up ever-larger portions of provincial budgets?

The idea that health care costs are rising to the point that they push out other priorities is worth direct attention. We've recognized the importance of the determinants of health, of education, housing, and so on. If health care costs are so great as to make spending on other priorities impossible, that's unacceptable. Fortunately, it turns out not to be true. While there have been some fluctuations, health care spending as a percentage of GDP has been stable across the country since the 1970s.[5] The problem is not that spending has risen, it's that revenues have fallen. Through successive tax cuts and decreased royalty rates the budgets of provincial governments have got smaller. When you decrease revenue and leave spending the same it's an increased percentage. The truth remains, as former Saskatchewan premier Roy Romanow said during the 2001 Commission on the Future of Health Care in Canada,[6] "The system is as sustainable as we want it to be." The question is whether the political will exists to change the direction of shrinking public revenue and investment.

This threat of unsustainability is the constant, and most compelling, cry of those who would establish a private health care system in parallel to Medicare. Driven by the belief that health care is a commodity that can be best delivered through profit, they argue that the current system would be helped and not threatened by this change. The evidence is clear: this is rubbish. Wherever it has been tried (in other countries and in limited ways here in Canada), a parallel system has increased waiting lists and practitioner shortages in the public system. It also erodes commitment to funding the public system by those who can afford to sidestep the queues, ultimately leading to two systems that are very different in quality and cost. This argument, and the body of evidence that supports not moving in the direction of privatization, is worth an entire book to itself — and there are many works to that effect, such as the Romanow Report itself, as well as popular works like Maude Barlow's *Profit Is Not The Cure.*[7] However, getting stuck on the ground of defending the current system is a trap of which we should be very cautious.

Too often, the threat of privatization has forced those who know the superiority of a single-payer, publicly funded health care system to become defensive. We find ourselves entrenched in our positions and sticking up for the status quo. To build a healthy society, and to move out of this defensive position, we must stop defending Medicare. We must look to expand and improve our universal coverage.

One of the first steps is to realize just how little of our health care actually is public. Commentators on Medicare often compare the Canadian system to North Korea and Cuba, saying those are the only other countries in which there is no private health care. While a provocative point, it's also a joke. The only part of our system that is really publicly funded is hospital and physician services. Everything else is a mix of private and public, with the lion's share being private. In fact, when compared with other OECD countries, Canada actually has a far lower proportion of public funding in key areas. For example, while over ninety per cent of physician and hospital services are publicly funded, only thirty-nine per cent of pharmaceuticals and five per cent of dental services are publicly funded. By way of comparison, the German government funds seventy-four per cent of drug costs and sixty-one per cent of dental care. Our overall public spending on health care, at about seventy per cent, is near the bottom of the pack of OECD countries.[8]

The costs of doctors and hospitals, the elements of the supposedly unsustainable public health care system, have actually remained fairly stable in absolute dollars. This means that, as a percentage of total health care expenditures, they have decreased considerably.

The real cost drivers are those segments that lie almost entirely outside the public system. The largest culprit in this regard has been the cost of drugs. Prescription drugs are the fastest growing cost in health care budgets, both personal and public. In 2009, Canadians spent $30 billion on pharmaceuticals.[9] Many patients have said to me they can't access the drugs they need to manage illnesses like diabetes due to the prohibitive costs of multiple medications. There is a pressing need for a strategy to decrease costs for the system and improve access for individuals.

Getting in on the Action

This need is widely recognized, and has led to renewed calls to attenuate the runaway costs in this least-controlled segment of the health care system. There has been much discussion of how we should pay for prescriptions: individually, through out-of-pocket expenses and insurance plans, or collectively through taxation; whether all medications should be covered, or if coverage should be restricted to catastrophic costs or specific age groups. While this is important, an oft-neglected, related issue is the question of who makes the medications. Many are available in generic forms, produced at a fraction of the cost of the original manufacturers. Generic companies then sell the medications at a relative fraction of the discount, which is to say that the profit margin on generic drugs is very high.

Leaving aside for a moment who will pay for medications, what if governments made them?

In my home province of Saskatchewan, as in many provinces in Canada, there is a long history of successful crown corporations. They effectively and profitably provide essential services such as vehicle insurance, telephone services, and electricity, and sport provincially patriotic names like SaskTel or SaskPower.

Let's consider for a moment a hypothetical crown corporation that produces generic drugs: SaskPharm.

By creating SaskPharm, Saskatchewan could provide essential medicines to its population, create local jobs, and save provincial health dollars. SaskPharm could produce and provide generic prescription drugs to Saskatchewan Health at cost, greatly decreasing procurement costs. These savings could be used for other aspects of the health care system, or reinvested into research and development. Prescriptions of SaskPharm products could also be sold to the public at a moderate profit. This would pass savings on to consumers while still providing operating and expansion capital. In addition, medications could be sold at bulk prices to other provinces and jurisdictions, along the lines of existing arrangements provincial governments have made with generic pharmaceutical companies. This would provide savings to other provincial governments while creating further revenue streams for SaskPharm.

The potential economic benefits to such an approach are many. A crown corporation like SaskPharm would provide jobs in research, medicine, information technology, commerce, and numerous other spin-off sectors, such as new markets for agricultural crops that can be used for medication production. The development of this economic niche could provide job opportunities for Saskatchewan's young, growing population and attract professionals and business people from elsewhere.

Should SaskPharm prove profitable in the production and sale of generic pharmaceuticals, there is also the potential for it to move into researching and developing new drugs. This is perhaps the most exciting aspect of this idea. Other pharmaceutical companies profit only through sales: if people stop getting sick, they stop making money. SaskPharm, as an arm of the provincial government, would profit by making or keeping people healthy. There would be a built-in incentive to create drugs specific to the health of the Saskatchewan people, such as new ways of monitoring or treating diabetes or helping to control the province's growing HIV epidemic. This would free up provincial funds for other priorities, as well as create potential for substantial profit with sales of SaskPharm original medications to other jurisdictions.

As it did with the introduction of universal health insurance, Saskatchewan could once again take a leadership role in health care by forming a crown corporation to develop and produce new medications. Saskatchewan tends to be an ideal place for this sort of experiment: its market is large enough to warrant the investment, yet small enough that change would not be exceedingly cumbersome.

Clearly, this sort of innovation is not without its challenges. The initial start-up costs, including market studies, establishing business plans, obtaining accurate scientific information and methods of production, personnel, and eventually building a production site would require a major financial commitment. Eventually, however, these costs would be offset by provincial savings in medication costs and the modest profit on sales to consumers.

The challenges are daunting, to say the least. Extreme care would have to be taken in relation to patent laws and trade agreements to be certain there was no legal backlash. Competition would be fierce, and we could expect bitter marketing and legal battles, though that would be attenuated somewhat by the lack of existing competitors in drug production in Saskatchewan. But these risks are no greater than those faced by our predecessors when introducing Medicare, which began in one province and eventually expanded to the entire country. This is a different time, to be sure, but there still exists an appetite for inventive, evidence-based solutions in public policy. SaskPharm is a home-grown way of controlling drug costs in Saskatchewan. It bears exploring. And perhaps CanPharm, and better health for all Canadians at lower cost, will be the eventual result.

Toward a Better Medicare

SaskPharm is just one provocative idea of how we can make the health care system more effective while containing costs. Others such as creative wait times initiatives, expansion of home care, wider dental coverage, and long-term care reform are important ways of innovating within the public system. Small scale efforts across the country have shown how changes to the current system can improve the quality, accessibility, and affordability of health care. What is needed is a scaling up of those localized success stories to a national level. On hopeful tool for this effort comes from Canadian Doctors for Medicare, a national advocacy organization led by Ontario family physician Dr. Danielle Martin. CDM's "My Better Medicare" campaign encourages health policy experts, clinicians, and citizens to share stories of innovation and success.[10] The hope is that these initiatives will spread to governments and policy-makers, leading to a health system that better responds to the needs of Canadians without compromising the integrity of the egalitarian enterprise of universal health insurance.

Of these initiatives, perhaps the most important and pressing changes to come are in the area of primary care. The innovations I described in chapter two — patient-centred care, interdisciplinary collaboration, evidence-based medicine, and social accountability — have been minimally integrated into day-to-day practice. We need to make the transition to the kind of care we need, and also the kind of care that is enjoyable and rewarding for health care professionals to provide. This will involve enhancing recruitment by valuing community practice. It will also involve paying family doctors and other generalist practitioners at a level more comparable to specialists and in a way that recognizes complete, continuous care over the brief and episodic. More than financial compensation, however, it will be the development of functional health care teams that ensure that each team member is working at the height of their skills that make the transition to primary care attractive and effective.

Above all, my point in highlighting various potential issues within the health care system, and initiatives available to improve them, is to point out that the system is sustainable if we want it to be. And that we should want it to be. In the chapter on growth and development, I discussed the necessity of some degree of redistribution in the face of dangerous growth in inequality. Medicare is an active and effective form of redistributing wealth. Those who have benefited most from our nation's wealth, and who in general have the good health to show for it, contribute to improving the health of those who have not. This is why Medicare is such a cornerstone of public policy in Canada, and a perennially popular one among the general public. It's also why it faced such virulent resistance upon introduction and continues to be under persistent, recurrent attack in the face of the overwhelming evidence for its success.

Those pressures and attacks will only continue to mount as income equality grows. The poor and disadvantaged use a disproportionately higher amount of hospitals, medications, and physician services. In Saskatoon, residents of the low-income neighbourhoods use thirty-five per cent more health care resources than middle and high-income residents, amounting to $179 million more per year in costs.[11] This makes it clear that health care is not the only way in which we should redistribute wealth. Not only does failing to address this issue raise moral questions, such as how to explain our willingness to help people when they're sick and dying but not to mobilize the resources to keep them healthy, but it also poses a risk to the political feasibility of Medicare. When we don't cover pharmaceutical costs or dental services, we increase costs not only for individuals, but for the system. As people are unable to pay up front, or if primary health services aren't available and accessible, they get sicker and present later in the course of their illness. Imagine the difference in costs between prevention of diabetes, or early identification and treatment, as opposed to long hospital stays and dialysis treatment when it was caught too late to prevent kidney disease.

A system as fair and compassionate as Medicare needs to reflect a society that is also compassionate and fair. If all the weight of dealing with the fallout of growing social inequality falls on the health care system, the cries of crisis will rise, and the commitment of those who are being asked to contribute more than they gain will continue to erode. Before long we will find ourselves in a situation where patients like Mrs. Peters or Brandon would be asked first not, "How can I help?" but "How will you pay?"

There is much that can be done to improve Medicare, but it must be accompanied by a concerted attempt to relieve pressure on the health care system by focusing on the rest of the determinants of health: income, education, physical environments, and more. This is how we can decrease costs in health care, improve access, and create the space needed to improve quality. Only by working on keeping people healthy can we hope to have a sustainable means of treating them when they are sick.

CHAPTER 8

Less Politics, More Democracy

It is only through such a system of global governance, placing fairness in health at the heart of the development agenda and genuine equality of influence at the heart of its decision-making, that coherent attention to global health equity is possible.

Closing the Gap in a Generation[1]

Change will demand the attention of all individuals, NGOs, business, communities, all levels of government and all sectors of our Canadian society. Success will require leadership from our prime minister and first ministers, from our mayors, municipal leaders, community leaders, and the leaders of our Aboriginal peoples. A whole-of-government approach is required with intersectoral action embracing business, volunteers, and community organizations. This will not be easy, but it can and must be done. We cannot afford to do otherwise.

Senate of Canada, 2009
"A Healthy, Productive Canada: A Determinant of Health Approach"[2]

Slow Walk to Democracy

Several years ago I accompanied a group of medical students from the University of Saskatchewan to Mozambique. We spent most of our time on the wards of the Massinga rural hospital, taking care of patients with malaria, HIV, pneumonia, and other serious conditions. Perhaps the most memorable experience for all of us, however, was far outside the walls of the hospital in the rural community of Tevele. For three days we stayed in the homes of members of the Tevele health *núcleo* and took part in a survey of mosquito bed net use.

Each morning the students would join their group for a breakfast of bread and tea brought from town, and tangerines fresh from the tree. They would then start walking from home to home. The groups, consisting of one or two Canadian students, two trainer students from the Centre for Continuing Education in Health, and several members of the health *núcleo*, walked for many kilometres. They crossed rivers on logs, tracked over hills and through brush, visiting all the families of the Tevele area. The families generally live in compounds of several small buildings with thatched roofs and walls of reeds or woven coconut palm leaves. At each house, the survey group would ask about who lived there, about what methods they used to prevent malaria, and whether anyone had been sick with malaria in the past year.

This survey was part of an ongoing research relationship developed between the local people and the Training for Health Renewal Program (THRP), a partnership between the Canadian International Development Agency, and the Mozambican Ministry of Health. THRP has worked with Tevele for several years to establish the health *núcleo*, the purpose of which is to improve the overall health of the people in the area. Early on, representatives chosen by the different *círculos* that make up the Tevele area met with THRP and identified malaria as their number one health priority. They then worked together to map the community and to perform an initial survey on malaria incidence and prevention methods. What they discovered was that very few people were using bed-nets to prevent mosquitoes from biting them and transmitting malaria.

The next step was the purchase and sale, at a low price, of bed-nets to people in the area. The follow-up study showed this to be quite successful. Many more families now faithfully protect themselves by sleeping under the nets, with pregnant women and young children appropriately getting priority use of the nets.

When we were doing the follow-up survey we asked those who had bed-nets where they had obtained the nets. Some said in Massinga, some from other towns, but many of them said "Canada." This confused us at first until we discovered that was what people had renamed the area under the big mango tree where the *núcleo* and THRP held their meetings. Community involvement at every step had resulted in adoption of and pride in the project. That adoption and pride resulted in changes in behaviour that are saving lives by preventing malaria.

This kind of community development work is sometimes referred to as Participatory Action Research.[3] The key features of this approach are inherent in the name. It involves research, serious inquiry into the causes of ill health and the means to improve them. The community that is affected participates fully in designing, directing, performing, and analyzing that research. Perhaps most importantly, the information discovered does not sit on a library shelf; it is translated into action that results in meaningful change for the community. The research, planning, action, and reflection involved in Participatory Action Research are laborious and complicated. It requires much revision, reconsideration, and patience on the part of the *núcleo* members and the centre staff. The end result is a community better prepared to tackle its own problems and health interventions that will work because the community believes in them. Seeing the *núcleo* members come out to work month after month is strong evidence of the dedication of the local people to improving their health. In Tevele it has resulted in better protection from malaria, improved local knowledge about HIV prevention, the building of a basic health post, and the income-generating Community Economic Development project discussed in chapter three.

The impact on the students was also significant. While far from the traditional setting for medical education, they learned more about the social determinants of health in the sandy yards of the homes they visited than they ever could in a classroom back in Canada. And unlike at the hospital in Massinga, where they saw only the sick and suffering, they met people at their best, at home where they are the experts. There they witnessed firsthand community strengths and weaknesses, and the role that income, education, housing, nutrition, and access to services play in deciding which families will thrive and which will suffer.

Democracy Diminished

These students also witnessed democracy — the rule of the people — at work: democracy in a form they had not seen before. The process of selecting priority concerns and the means of addressing them, led by the people most affected by the decisions, is quite different from the democracy we experience in Canada. Here the halls of power seem far removed from the challenges of everyday life, and often closed to the people whose lives are most affected by political decisions. This leads to disillusionment with the political process and cynicism about the people who seek election.

As a result, participation in elections at all levels is decreasing across the country. This does not mean that people are no longer interested in public affairs. In my travels throughout the country, through politics and medicine, I have been repeatedly impressed by the degree of knowledge, passion, and insight that Canadians have about important issues in their lives.

From big picture issues like international development and energy production to local concerns around the allocation of health care resources and community economic development, it's clear that people care deeply and want a say in the decisions that affect their lives and communities. The disconnect between passionate interest and lack of involvement stems from a growing perception that electoral politics are not a fruitful arena for public engagement. Be it the perception that the hands of governments are tied by international structures, beholden to large corporations, or simply disinterested in the voice of the average citizen, people feel they are being ignored in the democratic process.

Exacerbating this problem was a decision by the Canadian government in the late 1990s to eliminate the traditional door-to-door enumeration process in favour of a permanent voter registry. The fact that voters are not actively registered with each election has further contributed to decline in turnout, and emphasized gaps in participation along social and economic lines. In 2011, the Saskatchewan Party government attempted to add greater restrictions on the need for official identification and to remove the ability of First Nations band offices and other organizations to attest to people's identities for voting purposes. This would have particularly affected on-reserve First Nations communities, leading to even lower turnout from groups that have traditionally been underrepresented in elections. Fortunately, there was a significant outcry from the general public, the media, and First Nations, and this decision was withdrawn.

The issues of enumeration and voter turnout are extremely important, particularly for the governments and political parties that rely on the mass participation of politically aware citizens rather than the support of well-heeled special interests. When citizens feel their voices are heard they are more likely to be involved as party members, activists, and candidates. This brings fresh energy and talent to the political process, increases voter turnout, and raises the overall quality of debate.

No one understands local issues better than the people who live them every day. When decisions are made at a great distance, they lose the immediacy and common sense bred from local experience. In Saskatchewan, for example, there are over a million people, and at least that many ideas. There must be a means to bring them forward and put the best into practice.

What we need is less politics and more democracy. The only way we can hope to combat inequality and build a healthier society is through the meaningful participation of those most affected in the political process. A complementary system of distributed or participatory democracy would allow local people a more meaningful role in deciding their future. Rather than conflicting with our current parliamentary democracy, it would enhance it by helping counteract cynicism, increasing citizen participation in government, and adding value to our representative democracy. Instead of a revolutionary change of system of government, it would be an evolutionary change that reflects the ways in which — through population growth, mass literacy, and information sharing — society has changed, while preserving the foundations on which our democratic traditions are based.

Cotacachi

One particularly appealing model of such an evolutionary change comes from South America. Cotacachi, a city in the foothills of the Ecuadorian Andes, has developed citizen councils on education, health, the environment, democracy, and economic development. These open councils involve citizens from all walks of life in identifying key priorities and developing plans to address them. At the annual general council, they work together to determine how public resources will be distributed to meet these priorities.

The results of this participatory structure and process are proving to be remarkable. Infant mortality and illiteracy were identified as early priorities and have been all but eliminated. Electricity and sanitation services have been extended throughout the region. Perhaps the most important development is that citizens — rich and poor, Indigenous and European, men and women, young and old — are committed to working together to resolve key issues.

This model works because local and national governments support the process by following through with funding or changes to legislation based on the recommendations of the citizen councils. They also close the loop by communicating with the councils about which recommendations were followed, how it was done, and why.

The Cotacachi experience tells us that, given proper logistical supports and recognition from the existing structures of government, local areas can direct their own development. Of course, we cannot import wholesale a model from another context, but we can develop Made-in-Canada versions of distributed democracy. In Saskatchewan, for historical and geographical reasons, there is a strong history of community organization resulting in larger political changes. We have abundant natural resources and a small enough population to allow a high percentage of people to be personally involved. The development of flexible mechanisms, such as community assessment tools and staff and resource support for the organization of local councils, could provide the scaffolding for enhanced democratic decision-making. This would then set the stage for a debate that moves from emphasizing tough, top-down direction to involving people in setting priorities, planning how to meet them, and working together to get results.

Indigenous Knowledge and Guidance

Canada, like Ecuador, has a growing Indigenous population that has traditionally governed in a community-based and participatory fashion. The fastest growing segment of Saskatchewan's population is Aboriginal. Too often this is talked about as though it were a burden, or a challenge. I view it as our finest opportunity. Having a young, vibrant population informed by proud tradition can make us the envy of other North American societies.

It is an opportunity that is not, however, without its challenges. As a result of the multi-generational effects of residential schools and other abuses and marginalizations, First Nations and Métis people are unequally and unduly burdened with ill health, addictions, and poverty, lower levels of education, and inordinate levels of incarceration. Unless we work to change that gross inequality, that enormous and unsightly blight on our society, we will struggle to find a place for the coming generations.

There is no quick answer to these concerns. But there is an approach that is key. Too often in the past, experts have come from outside with answers that were simple, direct, and wrong, resulting in long term harm for First Nations and Métis communities and damage to their traditional lands and way of life. Good money has been poured after bad ideas, and the result is no change in Aboriginal communities and frustration on the part of the rest of the population. The answer to the problems faced by these communities is in the communities themselves, in their strengths, their traditions, and their ideas and innovations.

Taking this approach means going beyond narrow interpretations of the duty to consult to real partnerships. It means exploring innovative and controversial strategies such as resource revenue sharing and other means of honouring treaty rights and addressing persistent inequalities. It means working with leaders and community members to develop governance models and accountabilities that will make those innovative strategies successful. And it means working together to communicate clearly to Canadians, Aboriginal and non-Aboriginal, that ending inequality is of the highest national priority.

The only way to work toward a better future for Aboriginal people in Canada is to work alongside them. Communities will identify their own needs better than any outside agency, and they will also identify the solutions that will work in their specific context. This is no easy fix. It requires patient investment and the development of long-term relationships built on mutual respect. Given the attention it deserves, however, it will contribute to the long-term health and prosperity of the entire country.

So long as Canada is a country divided, it cannot truly develop. When we come to recognize the value of the contribution of all people, and in particular those long neglected and marginalized, only then are we on our way to building a healthy society.

Life of the Party

Political parties, the current vehicles for direct citizen involvement in politics, are often closed to the consideration of real change. It takes a moment of crisis, such as the misfortunes of the Liberals and the Bloc Québécois in the 2011 federal election, to allow the real soul-searching required to make bold decisions. The rest of the time parties are too concerned with electoral success, with appearing reasonable and electable to a sceptical public, to entertain truly novel ideas. The result of this inertia is the great divide between the converted few and the general public, with a great distance between the ideas needed for a healthy society and the political will to achieve them.

By introducing a means for more direct citizen involvement, we can build a bridge between communities, social movements, and electoral politics. Despite the criticism of the way parties operate, they are the most likely vehicle for this kind of experimentation. Let's take, for example, the case of the Saskatchewan New Democratic Party, the party I'm most familiar with and one that has recently undergone a major change. After governing from 1991 under premiers Romanow and Calvert, the NDP was defeated by the Saskatchewan Party (a right-of-centre coalition of disaffected Liberals and rebranded Progressive Conservatives) and reduced to twenty Members of the Legislative Assembly (MLAs) in the 2007 provincial election. The 2011 election gave the Saskatchewan Party a strengthened majority, with the NDP losing eleven more seats, including that of the party leader in what has traditionally been a stronghold. What has often been referred to as the "natural governing party" of Saskatchewan has been reduced to a shadow of its former strength, the worst outcome since the sweep by the Devine Conservatives in 1982. This should give both cause and room to reconsider itself deeply, a unique opportunity to experiment with democracy. For the Saskatchewan NDP, there have been numerous efforts in the past to renew the party, some (such as the famous New Deal for People under Allan Blakeney) more successful than others. The common flaw, however, has been the focus on a review or renewal effort, an exercise lasting a fixed amount of time. Only when the party struggles and threatens to die out are efforts made to resuscitate it. Once it is strong enough to win another election, its health is neglected and the cycle repeats itself. What is needed is a process by which healthy debate is maintained, where renewal is ongoing and constant rather than periodic and cosmetic.

A democracy is not a fixed and perfect system. It requires constant reconsideration to ensure that it functions smoothly and is truly representative.

Within a party, this would mean a continuous process of citizen engagement to keep it active and healthy. This goes beyond selling memberships and passing resolutions at conventions. Consultation can't be token and inconsistent; it needs to be constant and meaningful. A party that develops mechanisms by which to compile the diverse opinions of multiple and varied constituencies can lead the way in setting a vision for change at a larger level. Structures that enforce accountability of those in leadership to the party membership will strengthen the commitment of citizens to that vision. This could lead to the commitment required to develop functional local councils on key issues: the economy, education, the environment, health care, which is to say a meaningful system of citizen leadership in addressing the determinants of health. In this way Canada could follow the example of other countries that have been successful in enacting significant reforms and increasing citizen engagement. Local areas, based on local understanding and expertise, can work with provincial and federal governments to meaningfully direct their own development. The party that leads such a transformation would be a party that had truly found its voice: the voice of one who listens.

Leaping across the Divide

Change like this requires a leap of faith. We must trust ourselves and our neighbours. We must trust that, given the opportunity, we, the people, will choose what is best for us. The people can, given the opportunity, take the lead in building a healthier society. The challenge before us is to create the mechanisms to let those ideas be heard and put into action.

Unfortunately, such a leap of faith requires trust, a commodity in short supply in the current political climate. For many people — people who would call themselves proponents of democracy — the first response to such ideas is fear. They think that if ordinary people are too involved in decision-making it will be co-opted (depending on the flavour of their fear) by right- or left-wing radicals. The only way to get people to trust you is to trust them. It's also the best way to help someone become trustworthy. It takes risk, something hard to accept in uncertain times, but I believe that the frame of reference of the determinants of health offers us some hope. It allows us to set a standard to strive for based on common values. This type of framing is not intended to deceive and control. Rather, it is to stop the ongoing manipulation and fragmentation of the way we interact. The intent is to reorient our public discourse to the honest identification of common goals and the means to reach them. The common goal of a healthy society can be a means of bridging divides between people who initially seem irreconcilable.

Take for a moment the language of freedom. Enemies of the concept of the state, those who believe that government is a curse, often invoke freedom to advance that view: freedom from taxation, from regulation, from responsibility for the failures of foolish others. This freedom is like that of the adolescent who wants to enjoy the benefits of parental support without curfew or chores. This same child's parents, on the other hand, have chosen to bind themselves to one another and to their offspring, to support them and love them. Through this bondage they have traded immature freedom, which is selfish and hollow, for deeper freedom: the freedom to love one another fully, to embrace the challenges of raising children, to accept joyously the responsibilities accompanying their expanded rights. This view of freedom is also the attitude of mature citizenship, a citizenship that recognizes the great freedom that is represented by universal health care, unemployment insurance, secure pensions, a fair and compassionate justice system. The mature citizen asks the ancient question of Cain, "Am I my brother's keeper?" and replies, "Hell, yes, and happier for it!" For he knows that his contribution, needed by his neighbour now, not only does that neighbour good but also contributes to a system that will support him in his time of need, which comes for most. The next step in that freedom is not simply accepting and contributing to the common good, but becoming involved in its development. Populist movements, like the Tea Party in the United States, though often misdirected in their anger, have this at their heart. The ordinary person feels, correctly, that their interests and voice are ignored in the decision-making processes of so-called democracies. Honest intentions and frustrations are diverted from meaningful expression to angry demonstrations. There is a temptation, when faced with enemies that appear illogical and intransigent, to over-ride them with force or ignore them and proceed through trickery. The way back from culture wars, from the divisive and negative, is not less democracy. It is more, it is deeper and more open debate, it is the consideration of profound and complex notions, and it is the constant revisiting of core goals.

The above example is one where what initially appears to be a right-left issue, upon further exploration becomes far more nuanced. This is a useful exercise, as while that right-left split can be real on the one hand, it can be misrepresented and exaggerated on the other.

For my own understanding of right and left wing, I find it helpful and instructive to boil it down to two clear definitions of those political positions. At their cores, right-wing philosophy can be described as "every man for himself," and left wing as "we're all in this together." In terms of application, this is an over-simplification, but it's helpful to get back to first principles, untainted by words like capitalism and socialism, words that have been misrepresented and misused by opponents and proponents alike.

Advancing to a subtler description, we might say that the left emphasizes bringing out the best for all of society while the focus of the right is on bringing out the best in ourselves. At its best, the right encourages individual responsibility and initiative. At its worst, it blames and abandons the poor and breeds judgement and scorn for the less fortunate. The left, at its best, supports those most in need, and seeks to distribute the good of society equitably among people. At its worst, it fosters victimhood, mediocrity, and sloth. To paraphrase Gandhi, there can be no system that removes the necessity for people to be good. At times the far left is guilty of trying to do just that, of legislating utopia. At the same time, the far right chases a utopia of false freedom, abandoning the systems that allow people to develop enough to make wise moral decisions.

A view that balances the best of these two political philosophies is that we need to create the conditions for all to maintain a reasonable standard of living while providing opportunities for people to make good choices. The reason I choose to align myself on the left of the political spectrum is that while an attitude of "we're all in this together" has room to emphasize an ethic of personal responsibility and initiative, an attitude of "every man for himself" cannot provide for all and actively interferes with the need for an organized approach to improving society. The key to a healthier society is not the elimination of government; it is the re-structuring of government to be what it should be: a mechanism for achieving the will of the people, a truly democratic institution that allows the good instincts and ideas of people to be reflected in a larger plan. It is the idea of society as a project we're all working on, and government as the workshop.

Father Figuring

My personal motto has been, for a long time, be right wing with yourself and left wing with everyone else. That is to say, demanding of myself, insistent on hard work and moral rectitude, while accepting the weaknesses of others. With time, and what I hope to be some maturity, I've come to be more comfortable with my own weaknesses and failures, realizing that beating myself up over each moment of laziness or moral miscue was exhausting and counter-productive. I also came to understand, in life and in medical practice, that there are times when, for the good of the other, one must demand that they show strength and resolve. Sometimes you have to not help someone so that they can help themselves.

All this is to say that while I've arrived, conscious and committed, at a left position on the political spectrum, it's a broad spectrum. It is a search to do the good that works, a practical idealism. Similar to the toolbox approach to economic policy, what that allows is flexibility and the ability to recognize the ideals behind the positions of those on the "other side."

It is too easy, and happens too often, that we see people who disagree with us and assume the worst of motivations. Not only is this a shallow analysis, it also eliminates the possibility of finding common ground. Recognizing that, while you might not agree with the intentions of your opponents, those intentions are valid, allows us to move beyond hyper-partisan polarization in search of a common good.

My own approach to this is informed by my relationship with my father. Often while writing this book I have thought about how he would react. Wally Meili is a card-carrying member of the Saskatchewan Party. His political affiliation has always been to the right (and for as long as I can remember to the right of mine; I recall him describing me at eight or nine to a friend as "a good kid but a bit left wing"). He worked for Progressive Conservative Saskatchewan premier Grant Devine in the 1980s, investigating alternative markets for Saskatchewan agricultural products. When we talk politics we butt heads over parties, policies, and personalities.

If I didn't know him, I might see him as an adversary, as someone misguided and wrong. But I know better; he is a very good man. I've never met anyone who doesn't like Wally. He's generous, kind, and genuinely interested in people. He's been the model, throughout my life, of the good Samaritan, always helping people out of small jams and big problems. He's well-read and well-travelled, a successful farmer, and a dedicated dad. In recent years he's become a philanthropist, bringing medical supplies to aid projects in Central America and organizing clean water systems for Haiti. Beyond politics, we have a lot in common (sometimes too much; I frequently find myself sounding like him).

So when we disagree politically, we have to be careful. We can't discard each other's opinions, can't simply walk away and dismiss the other as a fool. Coming from a place of mutual respect, we seek out common ground, and the discussions we've had about the determinants of health have made sense to him. While I don't think he'll ever be a social democrat (though one of my great accomplishments in life was convincing him to join the NDP in order to vote in the 2009 leadership race), he reminds me that the "other side" is not so other as it seems.

Eddies and Loops

The need to look beyond our normal political circles and engage with those we don't agree with is important to remember as it paradoxically very easy, in these days of social media, to become isolated. The 2011 federal election is a great example. In Saskatchewan there were two NDP candidates who had reasonable chances of unseating Conservative MPs, Nettie Wiebe in

Saskatoon-Rosetown-Biggar and Noah Evanchuk in Moose Jaw-Palliser. These were thought to be close races and turned out to be just that, with the incumbent Conservatives keeping their seats by less than three per cent of the vote in each. But when I looked on my Facebook page, with nearly everyone's profile picture switched to an Orange Crush can and status updates full of links to stories by NDP organizers or in sympathetic papers, you'd think it was going to be a walk for the NDP. This happens partly because more of my friends vote NDP than don't, but also because Facebook and other social network sites track which stories you read and then show you more of the same. Rather than becoming more aware of what's happening in the world, users become more entrenched in their own beliefs.

With that kind of positive affirmation loop, people can become smug, assuming that any thinking person sees the world as they do and dismissing anyone who disagrees with them. Rather than helping them to reach their goals and serve their cause, it isolates them among a twinkle of activists, leading them to believe they're winning when they're only hearing the echo of their own opinions. This isn't to say that the use of social networks is terrible, just that they have their limitations and are no replacement for conversations.

For the good of all people, not just those on our list of friends, we need to take the conversation beyond local loops to include a wider audience. The way to do this is first to return to the language of health, language that works across divides of right and left, and then to take it everywhere possible: to churches and classrooms, union halls and company boardrooms. We need to risk ridicule on right-wing talk radio, not just stick to the CBC. This has to be honest — a real discussion with people, regardless of their affiliations. The purpose is not to convince the world of one set of solutions; to find common ground, we must first recognize that there is wisdom to be found among all of us. If I disregard the opinion of someone who opposes me, then I am the fool.

The High Road is Hard to Find

To many who've been through the hard slog of working for change, be it within the political arena or civil society, this all sounds pretty naïve. There are people in this game, some on what appears to be the other side, even more dangerously those who appear to be your allies, who will do and say things that are dishonest, mean-spirited, and manipulative. There's no getting around that. But there may be a way to get above it, which is to get over it. I say from experience that the more you take the bait, the more you worry about who's saying what behind your back, the more you risk getting sucked into the worst of the game. It doesn't have to be that way. If you can avoid descending into accusations and negativity about your opponents, if you can avoid mentioning them at all and stick to talking about ideas, then there is room for a different kind of politics.

People are frustrated by what they see in electoral politics. They see complex issues being dumbed down and misrepresented. They see childish bickering. They see scandal. They see politicians who are more worried about optics than vision, chasing polls rather than saying what they truly believe. They see growing division and self-interest replacing a sense of common good. At a time when more people are interested in the issues that matter, they are becoming cynical and apathetic about the process. Talented men and women who could be great candidates, who could lead the way to meaningful change, are scared off running by the behaviour of their potential colleagues and opponents. Many people are either turning off completely or contenting themselves with working for change on the margins while the mainstream gets polluted.

What I believe, and what drove me to run for the leadership of the Saskatchewan New Democratic Party when I did, is that the time is right for positive politics. There is a growing demand for something more from our public representatives. There is an appetite for a different approach, for candidates who are thoughtful and principled, who speak to people with sincerity, with genuine humour. There is a desire for what Calgary mayor Naheed Nenshi called "Politics in full sentences."[4] People want someone who can communicate with them about complicated political issues in a way that respects their intelligence, someone who doesn't dumb things down, but translates the issues into core concepts on which we can build.

Right now the low road is congested. Attack ads and scandal-mongering and behind-the-scenes manipulation are the apparent tools of the trade. Each party decries the dirty tricks of the others, but excuses themselves when they resort to the same tactics, pointing out the mote in their brother's eye and ignoring the log in their own. In such an atmosphere it's not easy to maintain a high road approach. But when ideas, notions of equality and justice, of a healthy society, are what drive people to become involved, it's easier. And it can work; it's where there is room for growth. The space is on the high road. The space is in appealing to the best in people, to hope and to dignity, to the forgotten notion that we really are all in this together.

Imagine for a moment a party with a plan to build a healthier society, a plan based on the evidence in favour of addressing the determinants of health. Imagine a party with an open code of conduct for its own behaviour, regardless of what the other side might do. Imagine a party that in opposition avoids cheap, partisan bickering but refers constantly back to the stories of real people and the issues that affect them. Imagine a platform that outlined the changes to be made in each of the key determinants. Then imagine a government that involves the people meaningfully in decision-making, judging every decision it makes not on short-term political gains but on the real impact on people's health. Imagine, instead of spin and opportunistic funding announcements, clear communication on the reasoning behind decisions, and elections that are truly based on whether or not the country has become a healthier place.

It's a far cry from what we see now, but there is room and appetite for such an approach. Taking the high road is not only the good and noble thing to do; it's also what will win people's confidence. If there is enough pressure to create a more equal, healthier society, then candidates will emerge who will speak this language. Our democratic system is suffering, and the remedy is not harder fought, more polarized politics. What is needed to build a healthy society is deeper democracy.

CHAPTER 9

Our Future Together

The impact of determinants of health and lifestyle choices is well known to governments and to health care organizations. Unfortunately, the key problem lies in turning this understanding into concrete actions that have an impact on individual Canadians and communities.

Building on Values: The Future of Health Care in Canada[1]

True prosperity comes from using the best of our abilities in economic and social policy to achieve the health and wellbeing of all people, rather than exhausting that health and wellbeing in the exclusive pursuit of economic wealth. Understanding the role of the social determinants on health outcomes at individual and population levels gives us a framework through which decisions can be made and measured. With the recognition that countries with greater equality do better in both social and physical measures of health, we have a general direction for how to proceed in reaching the goal of a healthy society. Sharing public resources equitably to improve the health of everyone is just and compassionate. It also increases economic productivity, public safety, and the quality of life for everyone, from the poor to the wealthy. It's the right thing and the smart thing to do.

Throughout this book I've explored some of the key determinants in detail, through the lens of real people and real policy options. This is an example of how a health filter, informed by the best local and imported sources of evidence, can guide political decision-making. Perhaps more importantly, this focus can serve as a way of realigning our democratic processes toward a shared notion, an identifiable common good. People care about health. They care about their own health and the health of their family. They also care about the health of society.

The core idea of this book is not just that health should guide our policy decisions; it should also be the language of our politics. Because people care about health, they are more likely to respond to political messages that reflect that concern. This is about framing, not in a manipulative way, but in a way that connects diverse and complex issues to a core concern. It's not an approach to advance the marketing success of one party, it's a means of rehabilitating a sick political system. A focus on health, demanded by an increasingly aware population, can force every party to reconsider its decisions and positions in relation to the determinants. It can establish an environment in which, rather than bombarded shoppers in the marketplace of clashing ideas and conflicting priorities, people can see themselves as part of a common project, as working together toward the goal of a healthier society.

> Another way to strengthen the social determinants of health is to support candidates of political parties that are receptive to the social determinants of health concept. Candidates who favour these ideas and the public policies that flow from them should be supported and those that currently do not need to be pressured to adopt these positions.
>
> — Mikkonen and Raphael[2]

Clinical Trial

This sounds great. The question is, will it work? As of yet, there is no large-scale, general election example of a campaign with a core message of a healthy society, based on the determinants of health. In Saskatchewan, however, there has been one small trial of this method.

After the 2007 Saskatchewan provincial election defeat, where the Saskatchewan Party defeated the governing New Democratic Party, former premier Lorne Calvert stayed on as party leader for just under a year. He stepped down in October 2008 to work for St Andrew's College at the University of Saskatchewan, setting the stage for a leadership contest. The race that followed featured an early front-runner, former deputy premier Dwain Lingenfelter, who declared his intentions in November 2008. With a significant head start in organization, funding, and name recognition, his presence put a chill on other candidates entering the race. In late January he was joined by Yens Pedersen, a Regina lawyer who stepped down as party president to run. Next came Deb Higgins, former provincial cabinet minister and sitting MLA for Moose Jaw Wakamow.

I watched this process unfold with great interest. It was an important moment for the party, as it needed to re-define itself after a difficult political setback and in the wake of the inertia that can come with a long term in government. I felt there was a need for someone who could help the party return to its original social democratic purpose, with ideas that reflected the realities of a new century. Supported by a group of friends and volunteers, I decided to take my cue from Virchow and try practicing medicine on a larger scale. In the first week of February 2009, I entered the race for the leadership of the Saskatchewan New Democratic Party. As the youngest, least well-known, and least politically experienced candidate, my chances were not good. I was banking on the idea that there was an appetite for something different, someone with a clear vision who was willing to talk openly and seriously about important issues. I also saw it as an opportunity to test some of the ideas I've been describing in this book.

From my campaign kick-off speech in February to the convention floor in June, I made the social determinants of health the core theme of my campaign. Speaking from the experience of a frustrated family doctor, seeing patients every day whose illnesses have political roots, I worked with my team to develop policy ideas directed toward the building of a healthy society. In every announcement, position paper, and blog posting, the notion of a healthy society was used as a framework. In the dozens of meetings and debates and leadership forums, from small town halls to urban auditoria, I came back, over and over again, to the concepts of the social determinants of health.

The first sign that this was catching on came from my opponents. We got to know each other quite well over those few months, and, over time, began quite naturally to borrow and build on each other's ideas. It gave me great pleasure to hear, after the first few debates, each of the other candidates start to talk about the determinants of health and reflect back the importance of policies that address these issues.

The second sign that this approach was working came from the public response to my candidacy. Rather than being marginalized as the Johnny-come-lately that, in many ways, I was, party members, new and old, welcomed me with open arms. Despite the inevitable gaffes of a first-time candidate, our campaign received positive media coverage and attention from online commentators. Donations came in steadily, hundreds of new members signed up in support, and the team of volunteers grew in both number and ability. As the final day approached, the common wisdom was that I was in second place and even had an outside shot at winning.

On June 6, 2009, the convention floor at the Brandt Centre in Regina was packed with excited members and media observers. Each candidate had ten minutes to present their view of the party's new direction, followed by which the members, in a one-member-one-vote system, would choose the new party leader. Those who couldn't be present had voted by mail or online in advance. After the speeches, and a tense round of chanting and sign-waving from the supporters of opposing camps, the results of the first ballot were announced. The results were just over forty-six per cent for Dwain Lingenfelter and just over twenty-five per cent for me, with Yens Pedersen and Deb Higgins receiving just under fifteen and fourteen per cent, respectively.

This result forced a second ballot, on which Yens chose not to appear. Instead both he and Deb chose to put their support behind me. This gracious show of support was appreciated and significant, but it wasn't quite enough to carry the day. After the second ballot, Mr. Lingenfelter was declared party leader with just over 55.07 per cent of the 9,130 votes to my 44.93 per cent. While it's always disappointing not to win, I was pleased and honoured by this result. At the start of the race no one would have predicted me being on the final ballot, let alone within a few percentage points of the leader.

There are an enormous number of variables in such a contest: the news stories of the time, candidate experience or political baggage, missteps or clever moves in campaign strategy, public-speaking style, and of course the hard work of voter contact and membership sales. It is my contention, however, that one of the major factors in this unsuspected success was the theme of a healthy society. Bolstered by the fact that it was delivered by a practising physician, this theme rang true to people. When I explained my reasons for running, they made sense, and more importantly, they spoke to something that people recognized as valid in their lives and the lives of those around them. All of us are intimately familiar with the impact of the determinants of health in our own lives; a campaign that addressed the immediacy and importance of those determinants resonated with people's own experience.

Shovels in the Ground

My venture in trying out this theme in a leadership campaign pales in comparison with another local social determinants success story. Despite the setback caused by the provincial government's decision to rescind funding for Station 20 West, the community-based organizations behind the project re-grouped, re-designed, and continued to work to raise funds. The politics of the decision and the need to downsize meant the dental clinic, SWITCH, and the West Side Community Clinic wouldn't be involved; the presence of some of the other intended partners was at risk, and the eco-friendly status of the building would have to be downgraded. Nonetheless, spurred on by the success of a Friends of Station 20 West Facebook group that garnered thousands of members in the days following the announcement of the loss of funding, along with a tremendous show of support at the community rally, the organizers committed to raising the money needed to start construction of this more modest version of the original plan. Volunteers put on dozens of fundraisers, distributed change jars to area businesses, held bake sales and buy-a-brick sponsorship campaigns. The City of Saskatoon sold the land to the project for a dollar, and early support came in the form of donations and mortgage guarantees from public sector unions and a local Credit Union. At the end of 2010, an ecumenical group of ten Christian church communities committed to raising funds within their congregations during the Christmas season in support of the Good Food Junction grocery store.

The board had learned of the loss of government support for the project on Easter weekend, 2008. After three years of struggle, with prospects for success looking very dim at times, the board learned of a large donation from Saskatoon philanthropist Joe Remai on Easter weekend, 2011. With another large donation from the Kinsmen Foundation of Saskatoon shortly afterward, enough money had been raised to start construction. Accompanied by a troupe of older activists who call themselves the Raging Grannies singing "Shovels in the Ground" (to the tune of "Bringing in the Sheaves"), dozens of community members and supporters came to the construction site to celebrate the successful campaign and applaud a ceremonial sod-turning on a rainy day in July, 2011. Construction of the community development centre is expected to be completed in summer 2012.

Some of the original elements of Station 20 West will be missed. I certainly wish our clinic could be alongside these other organizations. There are still many possibilities to work together in addressing the determinants of health, they're just that much more likely to happen when you're in the same building. Despite the disappointment that Station 20 West didn't happen according to plan, in some ways this is the better story. The issues of food insecurity and housing shortages in the core are better known by the people of Saskatoon. People on both sides of this often divided city came together, first in reaction to a bad decision, but then in action for change. The result is a project that is not only in the service of the people of the core, but will stand as an emblem of solidarity, a true community victory.

Escaping from the Phantom Zone

These successes show the currency that ideas of the determinants of health can have with the public. This idea is supported by the work of the Saskatoon researchers who first identified the extent of the disparities in health between low income neighbourhoods and the rest of the city. After that initial research, but prior to the release of their evidence-based recommendations to address the disparities, they did a study of community opinions.[3] They started by phoning 5,000 citizens of Saskatoon, male and female, Aboriginal and non-Aboriginal, from wealthy and poor neighbourhoods. The participants were asked about what factors determine health, about the relationship of income to certain health conditions and behaviours, what kind of interventions would make a difference, and what level of health disparity they thought acceptable.

The results of this study were largely encouraging. Though they overemphasized somewhat the role of nutritious food and exercise compared with other determinants, people generally recognized that income, education, employment, and other social circumstances have an impact on health outcomes. The people surveyed tended not to realize just how much income influenced the likelihood of suffering from certain health conditions or of exhibiting harmful behaviours like substance abuse or smoking.

While many of the survey respondents did not understand completely the role of the determinants of health, they did express a strong preference for more equal health outcomes. Most of those who had an opinion said that there should be either no or very little difference in health outcomes based on income. There was no support for the huge inequalities that exist today. Perhaps more encouraging yet, not only did people believe that the current inequality in health outcomes was unacceptable, they were also overwhelmingly (eighty-three per cent) convinced that something could be done about it.

So what we have is a situation where people 1) understand to a degree the role of the social determinants of health, 2) believe that large inequalities in health outcomes are unacceptable, and 3) think that something can and should be done about it. Despite this understanding and concern, for some reason the determinants of health and health inequality are not visible in much of the discourse of public policy. York University Health Policy Professor Dr. Dennis Raphael, a prominent author in the field of health determinants, describes the topic as existing in a Superman II-esque "Phantom Zone"[6] — powerful and important, but out of sight and mind. He goes on to implore advocates of public health to make the noise necessary to bring attention to the importance of this issue.

> Canadian research and advocacy activities in the service of strengthening the SDOH are so divorced from everyday public policy activity, media discourse and public awareness as to metaphorically suggest that SDOH researchers and advocates exist in a Phantom Zone of irrelevance.
>
> — Dennis Raphael[4]

What Dr. Raphael and other researchers recognize is the role that awareness of the power and importance of this concept could have on politics, on public policy in economics, education, environment, and ultimately on the most meaningful outcome: the health of our society and the people who are its fabric. The dual purpose of this book is to serve as a discussion of the need to share these ideas, and as one of the tools for doing so.

As a family doctor, my daily role is to take complex issues and translate them into language people can understand. There is a pressing need to do just that with the social determinants of health — to put them into context and clarify them so that people recognize just how relevant they are to their own lives. Hopefully, some of the stories shared here can bring this issue home for readers and spur them on to action.

Often when people want to create change, they focus on what is wrong about the current situation. I've certainly done that before, and to some degree in this book as well. It's easy, and sometimes useful, to point out the flaws in the current fabric. That will not, however, lead to change. In fact, a list of woes without a set of solutions can be paralyzing, leading people to feel the situation is too dire to do anything about. In the previous chapters, I spoke of a few different interventions that could improve the current situation. These include improving access to quality health care services and to education from early childhood to post-secondary training, addressing housing shortages and food insecurity in the inner city and rural communities, changing our energy system to stop climate change, ending the disproportionate incarceration of Aboriginal people, and using a range of economic tools to ensure that everyone can obtain the income they need for healthy lives.

These are broad strokes, and while I have pointed out some examples, they are intentionally short on specifics. The biggest impact will not come from any of my suggestions, but will be in the realm of democratic reform. If systems are introduced that allow people to become more deeply involved in the process of decision-making, they will demand a different approach. They will insist on decisions that improve the health of their families and communities.

This will not happen unintentionally. If people want a healthy society they must identify that as their goal, and take the steps needed to make it happen. This means connecting with those who are engaged in civil society and social movements. It means jumping off from the starting point of this book to deeper learning and understanding. It means joining — or forming! — a political party and advocating from within that structure for greater accountability and democracy. It also means the difficult task of talking to those who don't agree with you, of raising the uncomfortable issues of poverty and inequality and seeking common ground to address them. The idea of a healthy society, particularly one with greater equality, will certainly run up against many detractors. People will come up with all kinds of reasons why change is not possible, why we must only react to the economically inevitable, why citizens can't be trusted to make wise decisions, why we're stuck.

We're not stuck. There is a lot that can be done, and successful examples abound. We need to first see that we are all in this together. By seeing ourselves as part of a shared project, as working toward a common goal of health, we can create the environment for a new, positive politics. We can establish a functioning means of engaging our challenges and measuring our success in meeting them. This can enable us to improve our meaningful outcomes, to live safer, longer, and happier lives, to enjoy life in a truly health society. It can enable us to build our future, together.

References

Notes to Preface

1   A. Clarkson, *Norman Bethune* (Canada: Penguin Group, 2009).

Notes to Chapter 1: A Healthy Society

1   Commission on the Social Determinants of Health, *Closing the Gap in a Generation: Health equity through action on the social determinants of health*. Final report of the Commission on the Social Determinants of Health (Geneva: World Health Organization, 2008), p. 3.

2   S. Nettleton, "Surveillance, Health Promotion and the Formation of a Risk Identity," in M. Sidell, L. Jones, J. Katz, and A. Peberdy (Eds.), *Debates and Dilemmas in Promoting Health* (London: Open University Press, 1997), pp. 314-24.

3   Canadian Institute for Health Information, *Improving the Health of Young Canadians. Canadian Population Health Initiative* (Ottawa: Canadian Institute for Health Information, 2005).

4   D. Raphael, *Social Determinants of Health: Canadian Perspectives*, 2nd Ed. (Toronto: Canadian Scholars' Press, 2009), p. 7.

5   M. Lemstra, C. Neudorf, and J. Opondo, "Health disparity by neighbourhood income," *Canadian Journal of Public Health* (2006) 97: 435-39.

6   World Health Organization, 1948; https://apps.who.int/aboutwho/en/definition.html.

7   R. Wilkinson and K. Pickett, *The Spirit Level: Why More Equal Societies Almost Always Do Better* (London: Allen Lane, 2009).

8   Editor's Choice, "The Big Idea," *British Medical Journal*, 312, 7037 (April 20, 1996); http://bmj.bmjjournals .com/cgi/content/full/312/7037/0.

9   Commission on the Social Determinants of Health, *Closing the Gap in a Generation*, p. 116.

10   UN Commission on Human Rights, 1948; www.un.org/en/documents/udhr/.

Notes to Chapter 2: Medicine on a Larger Scale

1   R. Virchow, *Collected Essays on Public Health and Epidemiology* (Cambridge, UK: Science History Publications, 1848/1985).

2   *Ibid.*

3   M. Stewart et al., *Patient-Centered Medicine: Transforming the Clinical Method* (London: Sage Publications, 1995.)

4   C. Boelen and J. E. Heck, *Defining and Measuring Social Accountability of Medical Schools* (Geneva: World Health Organization, 1995).

5   G. Guyatt et al., Evidence-Based Medicine Working Group: "Evidence-based Medicine. A new approach to teaching the practice of medicine," JAMA (1992) 268: 2420-25.

6   www.rxfiles.ca.

7   M. Lemstra and C. Neudorf, *Health Disparity in Saskatoon: Analysis to Intervention* (Saskatoon: Saskatoon Health Region, 2008.)

8   Virchow, *Collected Essays*.

9   Commission on the Social Determinants of Health, *Closing the Gap in a Generation: Health equity through action on the social determinants of health*. Final report of the Commission on the Social Determinants of Health (Geneva: World Health Organization, 2008), p. 10.

Notes to Chapter 3: Growth and Development

1   J. Mikkonen and D. Raphael, *Social Determinants of Health: The Canadian Facts* (Toronto: York University School of Health Policy and Management, 2010), p.12.

2   D. Raphael, *Social Determinants of Health: Canadian Perspectives*, 2nd Ed. (Toronto: Canadian Scholars Press, 2009), p. 9.

3   R. F. Kennedy, "Remarks at the University of Kansas, March 18, 1968"; www.jfklibrary.org/Research/Ready-Reference/RFK-Speeches/Remarks-of-Robert-F-Kennedy-at-the-University-of-Kansas-March-18-1968.aspx .

4   J. Heath, *Filthy Lucre: Economics for People Who Hate Capitalism* (Toronto: Harper Collins, 2009).

5   GPI Atlantic, "The Genuine Progress Index: A Better Set of Tools" (Sept. 14, 2007); www.gpiatlantic.org/gpi.htm.

6   Canadian Index of Wellbeing; http://ciw.ca/en/.

7   M. Lemstra, C. Neudorf, and J. Opondo, "Health Disparity by Neighbourhood Income," *Canadian Journal of Public Health* (2006) 97: 435-39.

8   Canadian Housing Observer, "Housing Market Indicators, Canada, Provinces, and Metropolitan Areas, 1990 – 2009," Canada Mortgage and Housing Corporation; www.cmhc.ca/en/corp/about/cahoob/index.cfm.

9   *Ibid.*

10 P. Gingrich, *Boom and Bust: The Growing Income Gap in Saskatchewan* (Ottawa: Canadian Centre for Policy Alternatives, 2009).

11 *Ibid.*

12 E. W. Kierans, *Globalism and the Nation State*, The Lost Massey Lectures (Toronto: House of Anansi Press, 2007), p. 258.

13 J. Székács Jacobi, *Selected Writings by Paracelsus* (Princeton: Bollingen Foundation Collection, 1995), p. 63.

14 *Healthy People, Healthy Performance, Healthy Profits: The Case for Business Action on the Socio-Economic Determinants of Health* (Conference Board of Canada, 2008).

15 Holzer et al, Task Force on Poverty of the Center for American Progress, *The Economic Costs of Poverty in the United States: Subsequent Effects of Children Growing Up Poor,* April 2007.

16 *The Cost of Poverty: An Analysis of the Economic Costs of Poverty in Ontario.* Ontario Association of Food Banks. www.oafb.ca/assets/pdfs/CostofPoverty.pdf.

17 Commission on the Social Determinants of Health, *Closing the Gap in a Generation: Health equity through action on the social determinants of health.* Final report of the Commission on the Social Determinants of Health (Geneva: World Health Organization, 2008), p. 35.

18 "You know, there's two schools in economics on this, one is that there are some good taxes and the other is that no taxes are good taxes. I'm in the latter category. I don't believe any taxes are good taxes." Prime Minister Stephen Harper, interview in the *Globe and Mail,* July 2010.

19 Mackenzie and Shillington, *Canada's Quiet Bargain: The Benefits of Public Spending* (Canadian Centre for Policy Alternatives, 2009).

20 CBC News, *Lorne Calvert wraps up career in legislature* (May, 2009); www.cbc.ca/news/canada/saskatchewan/story/2009/05/14/calvert-final-day.html.

Notes to Chapter 4: The World Around Us

1   J. Mikkonen and D. Raphael, *Social Determinants of Health: The Canadian Facts* (Toronto: York University School of Health Policy and Management, 2010), p. 29.

2   J. D. Hulchanski, *Housing Policy for Tomorrow's Cities* (Ottawa: Canadian Policy Research Networks, 2002).

3 Federation of Canadian Municipalities, *Sustaining the Momentum: Recommendations for a National Action Plan on Housing and Homelessness* (Ottawa, 2008), p. 12.

4 Food and Nutrition Surveillance, *Household Insecurity in Canada*; www.hc-sc.gc.ca.

5 *Ibid.*, Aboriginal Status.

6 Hunger Count 2010; http://foodbankscanada.ca/hungercount.

7 *Ibid.*

8 Elaine Power, "It's time to close Canada's food banks" (*Globe and Mail*, July 25, 2010).

9 Joel Novek, *CED Food Initiatives in Inner City Saskatoon and Winnipeg: Very Much Alive at the Twenty Year Mark* (Canadian Centre for Policy Alternatives, 2009.)

10 Agrarian Reform; http://www.fao.org/righttofood/KC/downloads/vl/docs/AH264.pdf.

11 Environment Canada, *National Inventory Report 1990–1996: Greenhouse Gas Sources and Sinks in Canada. The Canadian Government's Submission to the UN Framework on Climate Change* (Government of Canada, April, 2008) 540 (Annex 10).

Notes to Chapter 5: The Equality of Mercy

1 "Ex-Posse kingpin turns life around." *Saskatoon StarPhoenix*, Aug. 28, 2010.

2 K. Healy and R. Green, *Tough on Kids: Rethinking Approaches to Youth Justice* (Saskatoon: Purich Publishing, 2003), p.15.

3 *Aboriginal People over-represented in Saskatchewan prisons.* Statistics Canada. *Canada Year Book*; www41.statcan.ca/2006/2693/ceb2693_002-eng.htm.

4 Fyodor Dostoevsky, *The House of the Dead*, 1862.

5 CBC News, "Canada's prison farm system being phased out"; www.cbc.ca/news/canada/ottawa/story/2009/02/25/prison-farms.html.

6 D. Cayley, *The Expanding Prison: The Crisis in Crime and Punishment and the Search for Alternatives* (Toronto: Tortontons Press, 1998).

7 International Centre for Prison Studies, *World Prison Brief*; www.prisonstudies.org.

8 R. G. Wilkinson and K. Pickett, *The Spirit Level: Why More Equal Societies Almost Always Do Better* (London: Allen Lane, 2009).

9   D. Calverley, "Adult Correctional Services in Canada 2008/2009," *Juristat* (Fall 2010), Vol. 30, No. 3; www.statcan.gc.ca/pub/85-002-x/2010003/article/11353-eng.pdf.

10   *Ibid.*

11   P. Smith, C. Goggin, and P. Gendreau, "The Effects of Prison Sentences and Intermediate Sanctions on Recidivism: General Effects and Individual Differences," *User Report 2002-01* (Ottawa: Solicitor General Canada, 2002).

12   International Centre for Prison Studies, *World Prison Brief.*

13   ChartsBin, Current Worldwide Homicide/Murder Rate; http://chartsbin.com/view/1454.

14   A. Ledding, quoting K. Healy, *Getting Tough on Crime the Wrong Focus: Weighill* (April, 2010); www.prairiemessenger.ca/04_14_2010/crime_04_14_10.html.

15   Author conversation with K. Healy, Saskatoon legal aid lawyer and author of *Tough on Kids: Rethinking Approaches to Youth Justice.*

16   *Supra* note 14.

17   *Ibid.*

18   *Ibid.*

19   CBC News, "There is an election on, isn't it time we talked? Guest column: National Chief Shawn Atleo on First Nation concerns"; www.cbc.ca/news/canada/story/2011/04/13/cv-election-atleo-oped.html.

20   A Ledding, quoting C. Weighill, *Getting Tough on Crime the Wrong Focus: Weighill.*

Notes to Chapter 6: Learning to Live

1   *Life and Works of Horace Mann*, Vol. III. Mary Mann (Ed.) (Boston: Walker, Fuller and Co. 1868), p. 669.

2   *Shannen's Dream;* www.fncfcs.com/shannensdream/about-shannen.

3   C. Angus, *What If They Declared an Emergency and No One Came?* Nov. 2011; www.huffingtonpost.ca/charlie-angus/attawapiskat-emergency_b_1104370.html#s487209.

4   *K-12 First Nations Education Funding Fact Sheet.* Assembly of First Nations, 2011; www.afn.ca/uploads/files/education/2._k-12_first_nations_education_funding_fact_sheet,_afn_2011.pdf.

5   Roger Martin, "Who Killed Canada's Education Advantage," *Walrus Magazine*, Nov. 2009.

6   C. B. Koester, *The Measure of the Man: Selected Speeches of Woodrow Stanley Lloyd* (Saskatoon: Western Producer Prairie Books, 1976).

7   Joel Westheimer, "No Child Left Thinking: Democracy at Risk in Canadian Schools." Videotaped presentation to the Department of Education, University of Regina, Jan. 2010; http://vimeo.com/9054678.

8   J. Mikkonen and D. Raphael, *Social Determinants of Health: The Canadian Facts* (Toronto: York University School of Health Policy and Management, 2010), p. 23.

9   P. Kershaw et al, *Does Canada Work for All Generations?* (Vancouver: University of British Columbia, Human Early Learning Partnership, 2011).

10   *Ibid.*

11   J. Beach et al, *Early childhood education and care in Canada 2008* (Toronto: Childcare Resource and Research Unit, 2009); www.childcarecanada.org/ECEC2008/index.html.

12   L. Monsebraaten, "Quebec's child care scheme pays for itself, economist," Parentcentral.ca; www.parentcentral.ca/parent/article/1012855.

13   www.education.gov.sk.ca/SchoolPLUS.

Notes to Chapter 7: Heading Downstream

1   J. Turnbull, "Building a Stronger, Sustainable Medicare for Canadians," AFMC-AFS Wendell MacLeod Memorial Lecture (Toronto: May 8, 2011).

2   J. Mikkonen and D. Raphael, *Social Determinants of Health: The Canadian Facts* (Toronto: York University School of Health Policy and Management, 2010), p. 38.

3.   C. Boelen and J. E. Heck, *Defining and measuring social accountability of medical schools* (Geneva: World Health Organization, 1995).

4   R. Meili et al, "The CARE Model of Social Accountability: Promoting Cultural Change," Acad. Med. 2011; 86: 1114–19.

5   "Total expenditure on health as percentage of GDP." OECD Health Data, 2011.

6   Commission on the Future of Health Care in Canada, *Building on Values: The Future of Health Care in Canada*, final report (Ottawa, 2001).

7   M. Barlow, *Profit Is Not the Cure* (Toronto: McClelland & Stewart, 2001).

8   "Public Expenditure on Health as Percentage of Total Expenditure on Health," OECD Health Data, 2011.

9   "Drug Expenditure in Canada, 1985 to 2010," Canadian Institute for Health Information.

10 "My Better Medicare"; www.mybettermedicare.ca.

11 M. Lemstra and C. Neudorf, *Health disparity in Saskatoon: analysis to intervention* (Saskatoon: Saskatoon Health Region, 2008).

Notes to Chapter 8: Less Politics, More Democracy

1   Commission on the Social Determinants of Health, *Closing the Gap in a Generation: Health equity through action on the social determinants of health*. Final report of the Commission on the Social Determinants of Health (Geneva: World Health Organization, 2008), p.174.

2   *A Healthy, Productive Canada: A Determinant of Health Approach*, Senate of Canada (2009), p. 1.

3   G. Dickson, "Participatory action research: Theory and practice," in M. Stewart (Ed.), *Community nursing: Promoting Canadians' health*. 2nd Ed. (Toronto: W. B. Saunders, 2000).

4   C. Koentges, "The Campaign in Full Sentences," SwerveCalgary.com; http://swervecalgary.com/2010/11/05/the-campaign-in-full-sentences/.

Notes to Chapter 9: Our Future Together

1   Commission on the Future of Health Care in Canada, *Building on Values: The Future of Health Care in Canada*, final report (Ottawa, 2001).

2   J. Mikkonen and D. Raphael, *Social Determinants of Health: The Canadian Facts* (Toronto: York University School of Health Policy and Management, 2010), p. 12.

3   M. Lemstra, C. Neudorf, and G. Beaudin. "Health Disparity Knowledge and Support for Intervention in Saskatoon," *Canadian Journal of Public Health* (2007) 98: 484-88.

4   D. Raphael, "Escaping from the Phantom Zone: social determinants of health, public health units and public policy in Canada," *Health Promotion International*, Vol. 24, No. 2, Feb. 2009.

Acknowledgements

EACH PATIENT STORY IN THIS WORK IS TRUE in concept, but each has also been altered somewhat: the names and physical details are changed to protect the privacy and confidentiality of all involved. Whenever possible, the inclusion of the story has been discussed with the patients. The ability to share in the lives of so many people, in intimate moments of birth and death, illness and cure, sadness and joy, is the greatest privilege of life as a physician. These interactions continue to teach me about life and how to live it, and I'm sincerely grateful to all who have shared their stories, their strengths, and their vulnerabilities with me throughout my training and practice.

While most books show the name of a single author under the title, they are generally the product of many minds. *A Healthy Society* is an extreme example thereof, as I have leaned heavily and repeatedly on the advice and input of friends, family, and colleagues in its preparation. Much of this leaning was long before there was any thought of producing a book. Rather, it was the countless classes, long walks, road trips, phone conversations, recommended readings, and fiery debates in which ideas and opinions were formed, smashed, and re-shaped. To thank everyone who was and is a part of that process would be a tome in itself. If you see yourself there, be sure that I do too.

As for the textual manifestation of that process, my sincere thanks to all those who reviewed the work in whole or in part and shared their advice. Thank you to Cory Neudorf, Erika Dyck, Max Fineday, Brendan Pyle, Noah Evanchuk, Peter Prebble, William Albritton, Doris Dick, David Forbes, Bill Peterson, Nazeem Muhajarine, Mark Lemstra, Jeff and Fleur MacQueen Smith, Father Les Paquin, Chris Gallaway, to my parents, Wally and Lea Meili, and to my oldest and most loyal friend, Paul Rowe. Deserving of special mention is Kearney Healy, one of Canada's finer minds in the pursuit of justice, for his substantial contribution to the ideas presented in chapter 5.

Going beyond the immediate contributions to the book at hand, I'm inclined to reflect on the development of my thought and practice on how best to work with communities. Looking back, there are some key role models who must be acknowledged. Fathers Don McGillivray and Les Paquin, through their work in northeastern Brazil, demonstrated how to live humbly among the poor and to work boldly for justice. The work of Drs. Gerri and Murray Dickson with communities in rural Mozambique has been an extraordinary example of honest and open partnership in pursuit of healthy development. Dr. William Albritton, Dean of the College of Medicine in Saskatoon, has been an incredible support and mentor in the development of my understanding of leadership and social accountability. Physicians who dedicate their lives to their patients — people like Chris Chandler, Stephen Helliar, or Stephen Britton, who have worked for decades with the communities most in need — have shown a practical path for the application of that understanding. All these role models have demonstrated what it means to be led by the communities we serve rather than trying to change them as we see fit. I don't expect to live up to these examples, but they set the standard for which to strive.

Two men of letters have had an enormous influence on my writing in general and this work in particular. Darren Dyck and Dave Mitchell are writers and editors of great talent and I'm lucky to have them as friends. Their input has been instrumental, as has that of Olin Valby, who has a great instinct for using story to bring an idea to life.

Karen Bolstad and Don Purich have taken a leap of faith in publishing a first-time author, and have been extremely supportive in working together to make the most of this project. My thanks to them, to Don Ward for his insightful editing, to Ursula Acton for proofreading and index preparation, and Jamie Olson for her perception and perseverance in developing the cover design. I join Purich Publishing in extending thanks to the University of Saskatchewan for supporting this work through its Publications Fund.

I've been thrilled to receive kind words of support from writers, thinkers, and change-makers who have influenced me. Some are close friends, others admired from afar. Names like Calvert, Barlow, Martin, Yalnizyan, Maté, Ashton, Guyatt, Marchildon, and Raphael evoke images of commitment, knowledge, and wisdom deserving of deep respect. What an honour to have them share their enthusiasm for the ideas in *A Healthy Society*.

Roy Romanow's thoughtful introduction is a particularly high honour, as it was during the Royal Commission that I was inspired to join with a group of students to engage in advocacy in favour of Medicare. In subsequent years he's become a friend and a generous contributor of advice, and it was due to his guidance that I became involved in Canadian Doctors for Medicare.

Thank you for taking the time to read this book. If you think the topic is important, I hope you'll read something else as well. There is no shortage of well-researched and richly described literature on the determinants of health. Because of that rich body of literature, this book is also not entirely new. These thoughts have found their way, in one form or another, into the works of many. Two key pieces are *The Pathologies of Power* by Paul Farmer and the WHO report, *Closing the Gap in a Generation: Health equity through action on the social determinants of health*. This book also draws heavily on scholarly works such as the studies of Saskatoon researchers Lemstra and Neudorf as well as Wilkinson and Pickett's *The Spirit Level*. What *A Healthy Society* does is explore the ideas in a particular context. There is some reinterpretation or reshaping, some focus on political will and the necessary conditions for change, perhaps there are even some truly new notions, and at the very least, much that bears repeating.

I would also like invite you to take part in the conversation. www.ryan-meili.ca will host a blog and discussion page to which your contributions would be most welcome. More importantly, it is my hope that the topic of the social determinants of health, and of a healthier body politic overall, is something you'll discuss with others. Only by engaging all citizens in the process can we have any hope of building a healthy society.

The final, and foremost, thank you to goes to Mahli. Her love and support have been drawn on heavily in the inspiration for and preparation of this work, not to mention her patience. Sharing my life with her and our son Abraham is my greatest joy.

Index

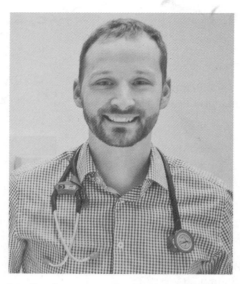

Ryan Meili is a family doctor at the West Side Community Clinic in Saskatoon. He also works for the College of Medicine at the University of Saskatchewan as head of the Division of Social Accountability, where he's responsible for helping ensure that Saskatchewan's future doctors are equipped to meet the health needs of the diverse communities they will serve.

Ryan is vice-chair of the national advocacy organization, Canadian Doctors for Medicare.

From its inception, Ryan has been involved in SWITCH, the Student Wellness Initiative Toward Community Health, a student-run, interdisciplinary, inner-city clinic whose mandate is to bring students from nursing, medicine, social work, physiotherapy, pharmacy, nutrition, and numerous other disciplines together to serve the residents of Saskatoon's core communities.

Ryan also runs the College of Medicine's Making the Links program, which gives medical students the opportunity to work in Northern Saskatchewan (Île à-la-Crosse, Pinehouse, and Buffalo River Dene Nation), at SWITCH, and in the rural communities of Mozambique in southeast Africa. One of the program's goals is for students to gain firsthand knowledge of the social factors influencing health by living among and working with diverse peoples.

Ryan lives in Saskatoon with his wife, Mahli, who is training to be a pediatrician, and their son, Abraham.